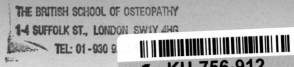

JENNY BRYAN and JOANNA LYALL

LIVING WITH CANCER

PENGUIN BOOKS

FOR OUR PARENTS

Penguin Books Ltd, 27 Wrights Lane, London W8 5TZ (Publishing and Editorial)
and Harmondsworth, Middlesex, England (Distribution and Warehouse)
Viking Penguin Inc., 40 West 23rd Street, New York, New York 10010, U.S.A.
Penguin Books Australia Ltd, Ringwood, Victoria, Australia
Penguin Books Canada Ltd, 2801 John Street, Markham, Ontario, Canada L3R 1B4
Penguin Books (N.Z.) Ltd, 182–190 Wairau Road, Auckland 10, New Zealand

First published 1987

Made and printed in Great Britain by
Richard Clay Ltd, Bungay, Suffolk
Typeset in 10 on 12pt Lasercomp Sabon

PENGUIN HEALTH

LIVING WITH CANCER

Jenny Bryan is a freelance journalist who specializes in medical writing. After gaining her degree in biochemistry and physiology at Queen Elizabeth College, London University, in 1976, she spent five years as science editor of the magazine *General Practitioner*, where she met co-author Joanna Lyall. Since then she has written for many newspapers and magazines, including *The Times*, the *Observer*, the *Sunday Telegraph*, *Woman and Home*, *Family Circle*, *Company* and *New Scientist*. In 1986 she wrote and presented a six-part television series about the use of everyday medicines called *Drugs for All?*. She also wrote a book to accompany the programmes, published by Penguin. Jenny Bryan has won two awards for her articles, which have enabled her to see some of the more remote parts of the world. Travelling, reading and music are her main hobbies.

Joanna Lyall was born in London and educated in England and Ireland. After graduating from University College, Dublin, she worked as a reporter for the *Kensington News and Post* and the *Western Daily Press*, Bristol, where she developed an interest in the Health Service. In 1980, after a spell on *General Practitioner*, she went freelance and has written for the *Guardian*, the *Observer*, the *Radio Times*, the *Sunday Times* and specialist publications, including the *Health Service Journal* and *Nursing Times*. She loves interviewing and is particularly interested in people coping with exceptional pressures. The idea of *Living with Cancer*, her first book, came from talking to friends.

CONTENTS

ACKNOWLEDGEMENTS

We are grateful to very many people who gave generously of their time and themselves for this book. In addition to all those who agreed to be interviewed on their personal experience of cancer we would like to thank the staff of BACUP and CancerLink, Dr Peter Maguire, Dr Robert Twycroff, Professor Tim McElwain and Joanna Morgan for their sustained advice and encouragement. Our thanks also to Margaret Wheeler for help in preparing the manuscript.

Chapter One

INTRODUCTION

The number of people who develop cancer in the UK each year – 239 000 – would, on their own, more than fill a city the size of Newcastle. One in three of us is likely to develop cancer at some time, and one in five die from it. But many of our attitudes to this hugely common disease remain uninformed, superstitious, and extraordinarily ambiguous. Far from being able to draw on a large network of support, the person with cancer often feels frighteningly isolated.

We dig far deeper into our pockets for cancer research than for any other medical cause – even heart disease, which accounts for a greater number of deaths. But a diagnosis of cancer can still drive away lifelong friends and turn families into strangers. It is not unknown for people with cancer to be shunned at work in case they are infectious. Many still believe this disease is best left unnamed and undiscussed. Patients complain of consultants who will not allow into their departments a single leaflet mentioning the word cancer.

But cancer is not always lethal. More than 40 per cent of people who develop the disease will be cured, meaning they will have a normal lifespan and die of something else. And thousands more live and work with their illness controlled by a variety of treatments which are being refined all the time. Right now over one million people are living with cancer in the community.

While in no way underestimating the physical, practical and emotional burdens that cancer often brings, we believe these can be minimized by knowing what to expect and where to go for help. There are few situations that cannot be eased, given appropriate support.

Coping with cancer is a highly individual affair. But there is no reason for it to be done in ignorance or isolation.

Our aim has been to bring together as much information as possible in a form likely to prove useful to people with cancer and their families.

We have tried to answer many of the questions about diagnosis and treatment of cancer which are often left unasked in the rush of the busy out-patients' clinic. We believe that people should be able to play a part in decisions about how their illness is to be managed, but this is only possible when they are fully aware of the options.

Information services and support groups for people with cancer – already well established in the USA – are beginning to take firm root here. And their number is increasing all the time. Our lists, though not exhaustive, are intended as a way into this growing field of support.

Our qualifications? Interest, concern and, we hope, a certain understanding of what it feels like to be told 'yes, it is cancer'. Neither of us has had cancer but we have seen three of our parents die from it. And we see friends facing up to this age-old disease with admirable courage but a disturbing lack of information.

We hope this proves a useful source for all those living with this prevalent, but still sadly secret, illness.

Chapter Two

WHAT IS CANCER?

If you thought that cancer was a 20th-century disease – a product of bad living, polluted air and over-indulgence – you'd be wrong. Cancer got its name over 400 years before the birth of Christ when Greek doctors, noticing its tendency towards sideways movement, named it after the crab. In the centuries that followed the disease was attributed to an imbalance of the four 'humours' which were supposed to keep the body in good health. The villain of the piece was the so-called 'black bile' which was thought to be produced in excessive amounts in cancer. It was as late as the 17th century before the black bile theory bit the dust, only to be replaced by numerous other equally far-fetched ideas.

Progress was inhibited by the fact that cancer is not one disease. There are over 200 different types of cancer and, although they share the same basic characteristics, they strike at different age-groups, progress in different ways and respond differently to treatment.

It isn't all lumps which are cancerous; in fact most are benign. The word tumour strikes terror into the hearts of most of us. Yet it refers to a lump or swelling anywhere in the body and does not necessarily mean cancer. You may also hear doctors refer to tumours as neoplasms; again this does not necessarily mean cancer. There are benign lumps such as cysts which are filled with fluid, discarded tissue or even hair. Then there are lumps of fibrous tissue – the stuff used for making scars, for example – which are called fibromas, and there are other benign growths made from glandular tissue, called adenomas. Many people have had lumps of fat, called lipomas, removed from under their skin.

Benign growths cannot be ignored. Most will stay harmless, but some can progress to cancerous tumours and so, in general, doctors prefer to remove cysts, adenomas, fibromas, and lipomas unless they are in such a tricky position that this is impractical.

On rare occasions benign tumours can still kill, even without becoming malignant. Meningiomas, for example, are brain tumours which do not spread to other organs like malignant tumours, but as they grow they press on other brain tissue eventually causing irreparable damage. Sometimes they can be removed surgically but only if surgeons can get at them.

BENIGN OR MALIGNANT?

In addition to their differences in structure one of the most important distinctions between benign and malignant tumours is that benign tumours stay put but malignant ones can spread. And it is the spreading of tumours which is the dangerous part. A cancer starts in a particular tissue, but few people die as a result of this initial 'primary' tumour. Most die as a result of the effects of tumours which have spread and caused 'secondary' tumours, also called metastases. These are found most commonly in vital organs such as the brain and liver; once there, they are very difficult to remove and they simply take over so that the organ cannot carry out its own vital function.

That does not mean that all malignant tumours kill, as the 40–50 per cent of people who survive cancer would testify. It is just that, having recognized that a tumour is malignant and does have the power to kill, it is very important to treat it.

Malignant tumours generally grow more quickly than benign ones. They steadily expand into the tissues immediately surrounding the initial tumour and then most malignant tumours head for the nearest bunch of lymph nodes. These nodes are like railway stations in a transport network which carries fluid around the body. A large proportion of our tissues is water. And just as arteries and veins carry blood around the body, the lymph ducts transport water through the tissues. Too much water and the lymph nodes get rid of it, too little and they see that levels are topped up. Also, part of their job is to get rid of invading organisms, so lymphatic tissue produces some of the cells of the body's defence system.

There are five main sites for lymph nodes – under the arms,

the neck, the chest, the abdomen and the groin. With such a spread they provide ample opportunity for malignant tumours to hitch a ride in the tubes which connect the lymph nodes and so spread to other parts of the body. But this is not the only method of transport. The bloodstream provides an even more important route by which malignant tumours can get about and reach other organs – often they will travel in both the lymphatic and blood systems.

Cancers vary in their ability to metastasize; cells may start breaking off and invading other organs quite early in a tumour's life or they may wait until much later. Preferences for new sites also vary, with abdominal tumours tending to head for the liver, breast cancers to the bones and lung tumours to the brain.

HOW NORMAL CELLS MULTIPLY

Under normal circumstances, there is a constant process of renewal and repair going on in the body. All the tissues of the body are made up of cells and it is here that the most basic and essential metabolic reactions occur. Each cell contains, at its centre, a complete blueprint of all the genetic material we have inherited from our parents. This is held in code as DNA (deoxyribonucleic acid) and is arranged in neat spirals to make up the chromosomes.

Every cell has its own life cycle which is a mixture of activity, rest and reproduction. Just how often cells reproduce depends on their function in the body; for example, bone marrow cells and cells lining the mouth and gastro-intestinal tract are reproducing all the time to replace dying cells. But some cells, such as those in the brain and nervous tissue, never divide.

Cell damage is not limited to the cell as a whole. It is not an all-or-nothing phenomenon whereby whole cells are either healthy and functioning or dead and disintegrating. Damage can be highly specific, affecting just the DNA, for example, and leaving the rest of the cell to continue normally. But because of the crucial nature of DNA, even relatively minor damage can have serious consequences. This is why the body has its own DNA repair mechanisms to put right any obvious abnormalities. Problems arise when either the damage is so severe it cannot be repaired or when the repair mechanisms themselves become faulty.

Damage to DNA can come in many forms. Chunks can be destroyed or deleted, bits can accidentally be cut out and reinserted in the wrong place or pieces can be duplicated. Although each cell has a complete set of genes, made up of DNA, they are not all switched on and active at any one time. It is a bit like a telephone switchboard; only some of the lights are on at any one time and just how many depends on how many lines are needed. Some genes, controlling routine everyday metabolic reactions, will need to be permanently switched on, while others will only need to come on for short periods for specific jobs.

Scientists are learning more about the mechanisms which control the switching on and off of individual genes, but they still have a long way to go. In particular, they have yet to work out the details of what goes wrong in cancer and why cells start to reproduce continuously to form a tumour. But in the last few years they have come closer than ever before to some of those tantalizing answers.

WHAT TURNS A CELL CANCEROUS?

Clearly, cells cannot be left to decide for themselves when to divide and regroup. In childhood, all the growth mechanisms must work overtime while in later life they must tick over quietly, merely carrying out routine repair and maintenance. It now seems that a whole series of growth factors are in charge of these activities – each with its own type of cell to look after.

But these growth factors do not just materialize by magic; they too need a signal to bring them on the scene. Some of them appear to be controlled by genes called oncogenes. This is not a very good name because it means cancer gene, and the reason they got this name was that initially it was thought that these genes and the growth factors they trigger are only found in cancer cells. It was only later that it was realized that both the genes and the growth factors are found in normal cells too. And oncogenes do not only control growth factors – they perform other regulatory work too.

What appears to happen is that in some cancer cells the growth factor genes get out of control. There may be too many of them or, instead of triggering production of growth factors as and when they are needed, the oncogenes remain permanently switched on. Either way, the result is a continuous supply of growth factors, which in turn makes the cells grow and divide with no thought of whether they are really needed. It is like a factory production line which takes no account of what customers have ordered. Goods keep piling off the line until they have filled all the warehouses and store-rooms and the packers have nowhere else to put them.

This is what happens when a normal cell turns cancerous. Out of control, it goes on dividing long after the ordinary needs for repair and renewal are met, either forming a solid lump of millions and millions of cells or dispersing the cells throughout the bloodstream.

Oncogenes and the growth factors which they trigger are a relatively new discovery, only made possible by the advances in genetics which have occurred in the last five to ten years. But although scientists have found some oncogenes and some of the growth factors, they have yet to learn exactly why normal oncogenes suddenly go haywire – turn on when they should be off or stay on continuously when they should be working intermittently. And they must also discover just how important the oncogenes really are compared to all the other factors that have been implicated in the cancer-causing process.

GETTING TO GRIPS WITH CANCER JARGON

Not content simply with classifying tumours as benign or malignant, cancer specialists have set up a complex set of coding systems which takes account of the type of tissue from which the tumour has arisen, its degree of malignancy and the extent to which it has spread. This means that you may hear your cancer described in terms which are at the very least incomprehensible and probably rather terrifying.

The word cancer is a collective term for all malignant tumours. A carcinoma is a malignant tumour which comes from so called 'epithelial' cells which line the air passages of the lungs, the inside of the gut and urinary system, provide the outer surface of the skin and make up glandular tissue throughout the body. But as this list shows, carcinomas or epithelial tumours make up the vast majority of cancers.

Much less common are the sarcomas – cancers which start in the tissues which hold the body together. That means bone, muscle, fat, tendons, cartilage and other connective tissue. Some cancers, mainly in children, are known to have started in embryo tissue. So they get the suffix '-blastoma', as in retinoblastoma, hepato-blastoma and neuroblastoma (eye, liver and a type of nerve cancer, respectively).

The specialists in hospital laboratories can tell a lot more than just the name of a tumour by looking at it down a microscope. Although all cells carry the same basic genetic information, they are adapted to the job they must do so their appearance varies. Thus a lung cell looks different from a liver cell; a bone cell differs from a muscle cell. When cells first start to become cancerous they look pretty much like normal cells. So a lung cancer cell will look like a lung cell, a bowel cancer cell like a bowel cell and so on. But as time passes and the cells get more and more out of control so their appearance starts to change.

Benign tumours bear the closest resemblance to the cells of the surrounding tissue. And, in general, the more malignant the tumour the less resemblance it has to the tissue where it started. Doctors call this differentiation. So a well-differentiated tumour is most similar to healthy tissue and is least malignant, while a poorly differentiated tumour bears little resemblance to its original cells and is the most highly malignant with, generally, the poorest outlook for its owner. There are a number of stages between well-differentiated and undifferentiated and laboratory specialists use these to tell their medical colleagues about the particular tumour they are dealing with. This is why doctors like to get a sample of a tumour – a biopsy – for examination in the laboratory.

As well as grading a tumour according to its degree of dif-ferentiation, doctors also 'stage' people with cancer according to whether or not the tumour has spread. A tumour can be localized – it has not spread – or it can be metastatic, in which case it may have spread to the lymph nodes, to other tissues and organs, or to both.

Doctors use abbreviations for these measures. Thus 'T' refers to 'local' tumour size, 'N' to lymph node involvement and 'M' to the presence of metastases. For example, you might see your tumour described as T2, N1, M0. That means it has reached a certain size, there is some lymph node involvement, and no distant metastases.

In addition to the universal TNM classification, different types of tumours are staged separately. Thus there are four stages (1, 2, 3, 4) to ovarian cancer depending on whether the cancer is confined to one or two ovaries, has spread within the abdomen, or spread beyond the abdomen.

These are the simplest forms of staging; there are other more complicated ones and if you see your cancer described in a staging code you do not recognize you can ask what it means.

THE FIVE 'R's

Once your treatment begins you will come across another series of jargon words, some of which are used interchangeably and mean the same. They can be very confusing if you don't know what they mean.

Response is what the doctors will be looking for in the first month or so after radio- or chemotherapy. If a tumour disappears altogether, this is called a complete response. If the tumour shrinks, this is called a partial response. Although doctors start looking for a response soon after treatment begins a response which occurs after three or four months' treatment is just as good as one which happens more quickly. Other words which you may hear are **regression** and **remission**. Regression is a vague term generally taken to mean a partial response to treatment. Remission is a term applied to people rather than to tumours. If someone is in complete remission then they are completely well, with no signs of a tumour.

A **relapse** is said to have occurred when the tumour of someone who has responded completely to treatment returns. It may also be called a **recurrence**. This does not signal the beginning of the end. A recurrent tumour may well respond to treatment again and disappear.

HOW CAN WE AVOID CANCER?

What proportion of cancers do you think are avoidable? Ten per cent? Twenty? Perhaps 30 per cent? You may be surprised to learn that some scientists now estimate that up to three-quarters of cancers could be prevented if we took better care of our health. The big unknown in the equation is the importance of diet in avoiding cancer. Numerous studies are underway to find out just how important diet is in contributing to cancer, and these results will swing the scales for or against cancer being a largely preventable disease.

Already well established is the fact that smoking is responsible for nearly a third of all cancer deaths. About 100 000 people die each year in the UK from lung and circulatory diseases resulting from smoking. As many as 90 per cent of the 40 000 lung cancer deaths are caused by smoking. And about 200 deaths of non-smokers from lung cancer are now attributed to the effects of 'passive smoking' – breathing in the smoke from other people's cigarettes.

There can be very few smokers in this country who are not aware of the dangers and while the proportion of men who smoke is falling it seems that women are finding it much harder to give up. As a result, it is expected that lung cancer will soon beat even breast cancer as the biggest killer of women in the UK. People who give up smoking do reduce their risk of lung cancer. Just how long this takes depends on how heavily they smoked. But even a long-term heavy smoker reduces the risk of lung cancer to that of someone who has never smoked within 10–15 years of giving up. As an extra incentive he reduces his risk of heart disease to normal within two years of giving up cigarettes.

Lung cancer is not the only form of the disease which has been linked to cigarettes. Smoking, especially in combination with alcohol abuse, is believed to play an important part in throat cancer and, more recently, it has been implicated in cervical cancer. Deaths from alcohol-related cancers pale into insignificance alongside the effects of smoking. Nevertheless, alcohol abuse causes about three per cent of cancers – mainly of the mouth, throat and, of course, the liver.

Dozens of occupations have been linked to increased risk of cancer, and asbestos is probably the best known industrial carcinogen. Now that so many of the risks have been recognized strict safety precautions are implemented where there is a chance of exposure to carcinogens. Some studies have suggested that the wives of men who are exposed to carcinogens through their work may be at increased risk of cancer, but further work is needed to confirm this.

Diet is one of the most recently implicated and possibly most controversial factors in cancer. There is no doubt that bowel and stomach cancers are more common in Western countries where people eat rich refined foods than in developing countries where diets are higher in fibre and lower in protein. People who are seriously overweight risk not only a heart attack but cancer too. Most recently, breast cancer has been linked to a high fat/low fibre diet, though this needs more research before definitive answers can be given.

For a growing number of reasons, it seems wise to shift the balance of the diet towards more fresh food and fewer calories. White meat and fish are probably preferable to fatty red meats; wholemeal bread, potatoes and pasta, fresh fruit and vegetables preferable to processed packaged foods, especially those with high sugar contents. This does not mean that any specific component of the Western diet is carcinogenic. But since fibre helps to speed food through the gut this may help reduce exposure to substances in the diet which may contribute to cancer.

There is a general move away from food additives, since some people believe that these may be carcinogenic in some way. There is little to suggest that this is the case but equally there is little information about the long-term effects – good or bad – of these additives.

Estimates of just how important diet is in contributing to cancer vary enormously, from those who say it contributes to only one in ten cancer deaths to those who put a whopping 70 per cent tag on it.

Still relatively new to the preventable cancers scene – at any rate in the UK – is the exposure to sunlight. The UV-B rays to be found in sunshine have long been linked to the high levels of skin cancer found in Australia. The fair skins of Australians combined with their prolonged exposure to intense sunlight have combined to give them the highest incidence of skin cancer in the world.

As more Britons take at least one foreign holiday in the sun, and many like to keep their tans topped up by using sunlamps all year round, so the number of cases of skin cancer is increasing. In particular, cases of the most serious form of skin cancer, malignant melanoma, are increasing. And although numbers rank nowhere near those for the commonest cancers the rate at which skin cancer is increasing is alarming. Scientists now believe that it may not be just the UV-B rays which are harmful but also the UV-A rays which are included in sun-beds because they have been assumed to be harmless.

You are not going to get cancer from the occasional half-hour on a sun-bed. And people with dark skins are probably at very little risk. It seems to be sunburn rather than sun-tan which is increasing the risk of skin cancer. So people with fair skins, or redheads, should use effective sun-screen creams before exposing themselves to UV-A or UV-B rays during sun binges either on the beaches of the Mediterranean or at the local beauty parlour.

IS CANCER CATCHING?

Many people with cancer report that friends no longer contact them; sometimes they are embarrassed but often they seem afraid that by associating with someone with the disease they are pushing up their own chances of 'catching' it. This simply is not true. You won't get cancer by sitting in the same room as someone with the disease, by touching or talking with them, even by sharing a tooth-brush. Cancer itself is not catching.

In a small number of relatively uncommon cancers there is evidence that exposure to a virus can lead to the disease. In the UK the most well known example of this is the link between the wart papilloma virus and cancer of the cervix; the herpes virus has also been implicated and may well have some role in cervical cancer, but recently the evidence has been stacking against the wart virus. For years it has been women who have been warned not to be 'promiscuous' for fear of putting themselves at risk of cervical cancer. But there is growing evidence that a woman should be at least as careful of her partner's sexual history as her own. She may have remained faithful to her childhood sweetheart, but if he has picked up the wart virus during some casual sexual encounter he will be putting all the women he sleeps with at risk.

This does not mean that every woman who has venereal warts will get cervical cancer. There may be small changes in the cells of the cervix, which return to normal, or there may be no changes at all. However, there is a possibility that the abnormal cells will turn malignant, which is why it is so important to have regular cervical smears to pick up the first signs of any abnormality.

Another form of cancer which has had more than a casual brush with viral infection over the years is leukaemia. At present there is no evidence that the vast majority of leukaemias have anything to do with viruses, but it could be that one of the rarer forms of the disease is caused by a virus.

Not of great importance to Britons but of great significance to Africans and Asians is the link between the Epstein-Barr virus and cancer. This herpes-like virus was first isolated from African children with a form of lymphoma, named after its discoverer as Burkitt's lymphoma. And it was soon realized that the virus was also present in people with nasopharyngeal cancer in South East Asia. Such facial and neck cancers are rare in the UK, but since the disease is so common in China and other neighbouring countries the viral link is crucial. Indeed, a vaccine is now being developed against the Epstein-Barr virus in the hope that both Burkitt's lymphoma and some nasopharyngeal cancers can be wiped out altogether.

A vaccine is already showing promising results in preventing liver infections caused by the blood-borne virus hepatitis B. At first glance this may seem of little relevance to people with cancer, but an estimated 80 per cent of liver tumours follow hepatitis infection.

So, strictly speaking, cancer is not catching, but the viruses which have been linked to some cancers are. Just because you catch the virus you do not necessarily get the cancer. All of these viruses are passed on mainly through sexual contact or through exposure to infected blood.

CAN WE INHERIT CANCER?

Cancer is not a genetic disease, passed on through generations like haemophilia or cystic fibrosis. Nor is there any clear-cut evidence of it 'running in families' like asthma or eczema. Some families do seem to have more than their fair share of cancer. But since one in three people do get cancer at some time in their life it is hardly surprising that every family has two or three members who have or have had cancer. This said, a few cancers do tend to occur rather more commonly within families than would be expected.

Breast cancer is perhaps the best known of these. A woman whose mother had breast cancer is at increased risk of developing it, particularly if a second close relation, such as a sister, has also had it. The familial factor may not on its own be enough to turn the odds against you. Other factors, including not having any children or starting a family very late, also seem slightly to increase the risk of breast cancer. So it may be that a collection of these risk factors, including a mother or sister with the disease, is enough to trigger the disease.

Doctors at St Mark's Hospital, London, which specializes in colo–rectal diseases, recently started family clinics for people worried about getting bowel tumours after other members of their family got the disease. Anyone who has two or more close relatives who have suffered from bowel cancer can contact the Hospital.

The family clinics have been set up because there is some evidence that a small proportion of bowel cancers may have some familial link. Not least, doctors want to gather information about families who have two or more people with bowel cancer to see if there are any common factors. And, where there are obvious dietary deficiencies which could put people at risk, they can give advice.

In addition to breast and bowel tumours, stomach and womb cancers do tend to crop up in families over several generations. It is not so much that they occur but that members of some families tend to suffer from them at a rather earlier age than would normally be expected. It is worth while being on the look out for early symptoms if your family does seem to be prone to a certain type of cancer and to let your doctor know of any family history of cancer. But it is important not to get worked up about it; you don't want to become fixated on the possibility that you will get cancer just because Aunt Sally did!

Some people may have heard of one rare, inheritable form of cancer. Retinoblastoma is an eye tumour which occurs in one in 20 000 children and can be treated effectively with radiotherapy. Some cases are inherited and so if there is any history of the disease in your family it is important to have blood tests to see if you could be a carrier and to seek genetic counselling.

Rather more common is an inherited condition which makes people develop numerous small growths in their bowel, called polyps. These in themselves are harmless but generally need to be removed because they can turn cancerous. And people who regularly get large numbers of these growths are often advised to have their large bowel removed in case one or more unnoticed growths become cancerous.

WILL I GET CANCER IF I GO ON THE PILL?

In 1983 two reports appeared in the same issue of the *Lancet*, one linking the contraceptive Pill to cancer of the cervix, the other linking it to breast cancer. Since then, research has yielded conflicting results. So just how serious are these results?

The main problem in answering this question lies in the fact that most women who took the Pill in the early days have still not reached the age when cancer is most common. There is no reason to expect an epidemic of cancers in 60-year-old women who took the Pill, but to pronounce the Pill entirely safe and without risk before a generation of Pill-users starts collecting their pensions would be premature.

Adding to the problem is the fact that all these women took the old-fashioned Pills which contained much bigger amounts of hormones than today's Pills. While providing important pointers to the long-term effects of the Pill, studies conducted so far are not entirely relevant to today's women as the smaller amounts of hormone now used are expected to cause fewer long-term effects. One new study soon to get underway in the UK will be the first to look at the effects of 'low-dose' contraceptive Pills on women's health. But it will be years before this and similar studies come up with the answers that women considering the Pill today want to have.

Evidence that the Pill may increase the risk of breast or cervical cancer has to be seen in the light of evidence that it actually protects against cancers of the womb and ovaries. Women who start menstruating at an early age and who have a relatively late menopause, particularly if they do not have children, run the greatest risk of developing ovarian cancer. This is thought to be something to do with the number of times they ovulate; the Pill, of course, prevents ovulation and so this may be how it reduces the risk of ovarian cancer.

Back on the debit side, a recent study confirmed what has been suspected for some time – that the Pill increases women's chances of getting liver cancer, to the tune of twelve extra cases a year; hardly a major source of concern to the vast majority of women in Britain, where liver cancer is relatively rare and kills less than 500 women a year.

The results of breast cancer studies are likely to determine whether the balance between the risks and benefits of the Pill are sufficiently in our favour for women to continue taking it for long periods of time.

In the meantime we must weigh up the benefits of the Pill against those of other methods of contraception. Barrier methods of contraception certainly help protect us from venereal infection and probably cervical cancer, but do not guarantee us free of the worry of pregnancy. Intrauterine devices are highly effective and on the whole are very satisfactory for women who have had children, but are much less acceptable for young women who are planning to start a family in the future. In these women, the devices may be painful and cause bleeding and there is some risk of infection and infertility.

If we decide that the risks of cervical and breast cancers are outweighed by the benefits of the Pill, then it is vital to have regular cervical and breast examinations to check that there are no signs of abnormalities, whether or not they are caused by the Pill.

How regular is regular? Current advice is that all women should examine their breasts each month, generally a week or so after a period. Anyone worried about any lump or bump should see their doctor. At present, doctors are only paid to carry out cervical smears every five years on women over 35. But responsible general practitioners, and family planning clinics, will do smears on all sexually active women. This means women who have ever had sex; it does not matter if you have no partner at the time your smear is due. Many doctors believe that five years is not sufficiently often and they perform smears routinely every three years, or even more often.

How long is it safe to stay on the Pill? If we had the answer to this question all our problems would be over. We could take the Pill during the 'safe' years and then transfer to another method as soon as the time limit was up. In general, women are advised to give up the Pill when they reach their late 30s to reduce the risk of circulatory problems – earlier if they smoke or are overweight. In theory it is young women still in their teens who may be at increased risk of cancer if they take the Pill. The cells in their breasts and cervix are still maturing and may be more susceptible to things which could cause cancerous changes – whether that means hormones in the Pill or viruses. Yet teenagers are just the group who need effective, simple contraception and may not use barrier methods correctly and regularly. Again, it is important to weigh up the possible but unknown long-term risks of the Pill against the all too obvious short-term risks of inadequate contraception.

The advice on any drugs must be 'don't take them unless you need them', and the Pill is no different in this respect from other drugs. Why put up with side-effects if you are getting no benefit? It must be apparent that for those who are getting immediate benefits there are no easy answers about whether or not it is safe to take the Pill. Each woman must weigh up the possible risks against the obvious benefits and make her own decision.

DO I HAVE A CANCER PERSONALITY?

Ever since someone claimed that people who get cancer are introvert and those who have heart attacks are extrovert we have all been rushing around trying to change our personalities. The extroverts don't want heart attacks so they've been taking relaxation classes and learning how to say no to their bosses. And

the introverts worried about cancer have been going on asser-
tiveness courses and learning how to be aggressive. What are we
doing to ourselves?!

Our personalities are a product of the genes we inherited
from our parents and the experiences we went through as we grew
up. And there is not a lot we can do to alter them. We can bring
out particularly attractive characteristics and we can try to suppress
the less pleasant ones. We all make New Year's resolutions to be
nice to people who really get up our noses, and we promise
faithfully not to lose our temper so easily when people we work
with are incompetent. But how long does it last? A week? A month?
Rarely until the next New Year's Eve.

Critics of courses which attempt to train people to cope better
with life – to relax under pressure, to stand up for themselves when
they are being put upon – argue that there is no evidence of long-
term benefits. The laid-back executives still get heart attacks and
the office mouse still gets cancer. Equally, we all know plenty of
dynamic active people who get cancer and recluses who have heart
attacks. It is just not possible to make cut and dried statements
about who will get the heart attacks and who will get the cancers.
Having said this, there is no getting away from the fact that we all
know people who seem to get a bum deal out of life and seem
somehow to bring it on themselves by their negative approach.

Time and again, when you read the stories of people who
write about their cancers there is a series of events which seemed to
lead inevitably towards the diagnosis.

Critics of the stress and cancer theory argue that since major
'life events' – a death of a loved one, loss of a job, moving house,
divorce – are so common it is surprising that we don't all get
cancer at some point. With over three million on the dole there
should be an epidemic of cancer. And they point out that for every
study linking stress with cancer there are two more which fail to
show any link.

Those who believe that stress does play a role feel that it may
not be the stress itself but the way that people perceive it which
determines whether or not they get cancer. One recent study of
women with benign breast disease or cancer showed that the
women who got the cancers rated the upsetting events which had

befallen them far more seriously than those who did not get cancer. So whereas some women coped with a death in the family, a divorce or whatever, for others their whole world fell apart.

But how can you translate stressful events into cancer? What is the bridge that links the psychological factor with the physical one? The stress lobby believes that it is the immune system. They argue that stress triggers the release of chemicals in the body which are capable of suppressing our normal immunity to disease. And, as a result, our defence cells no longer recognize and destroy cells which are turning cancerous.

It is a lovely theory, but immunologists continue to doubt whether the immune system really does have a central role to play in cancer. Why, they argue, if the immune system is so important, don't drugs which boost it cure cancer; remember the disappointment over interferon. And why don't more people whose immune systems are suppressed by drugs – not least those who are having anti-cancer drugs – get new primary cancers as a *result* of their treatments; a few do, but the vast majority don't.

Studies have shown that the immune system is suppressed after a bereavement, for example. But it soon bounces back. Widows and widowers do of course get cancer, but then so do a large number of older people whether they are married, single or divorced.

Perhaps one of the most damning things against the stress theory relates to breast cancer. Many of the studies on stress and cancer have been done on women with breast cancer, mainly because there are fewer other contributory factors than in other cancers to confuse the results. (You could not, for example, separate the stress factor in lung cancer because of the big contribution which smoking makes to the disease.)

The studies on breast cancer have tried to relate stressful events which have occurred in the previous 12–18 months to the subsequent development of cancer. Yet there is growing evidence that there is a long 'lag time' between the cell changes which lead to cancer and the appearance of a tumour. It is thought that the first cell changes may happen up to ten years before the breast cancer is found. So the damage is done long before any major emotional upset occurs.

To scientific minds, the theories relating personality and stress to cancer remain unproven. And, until someone can show that by stepping in and adapting someone's personality or changing the way they handle long-term stress you can reduce their chances of cancer, scientists will remain unconvinced.

Most of all, their medical colleagues are worried that people will be misled into believing that the theories are proven and will blame themselves for their own cancers. Already, they are seeing people who, as well as being depressed about their illness, are torturing themselves that if only they had been more positive and outgoing in life they could have avoided getting cancer. And that simply is not true. The case against cigarettes may be proven and there is good evidence against the Western diet, but stress and personality are still in the dock and the trial has hardly begun.

Chapter Three

TELLING PEOPLE ABOUT CANCER

'I found I wasn't expected to be angry and that upset me. It seemed I had every reason to be angry.' (Woman with extensive cancer)

'Thirty new patients a clinic . . . five minutes for each . . . it isn't easy.' (Consultant surgeon)

'It annoyed me when people rang up and started asking about the "growth". I used to say "you mean the cancer". I resented the implication I had something unmentionable. . .'

'The GP explaining my father was dying of prostate cancer did not hide how upset she was. Her father died of that too. I still remember the look in her eyes. She was very human.'

'I regretted all the times I had tiptoed around the bed avoiding a cancer patient's eyes, delaying explanations. I know how lonely it feels.' (Dr Vicky Clement-Jones, founder of the British Association of Cancer United Patients, on learning she had cancer)

HOW MUCH WILL YOU BE TOLD?

'Nurse, have I got cancer?' Faced with the question in the middle of the night the young student nurse obeyed instructions that only doctors could discuss diagnoses, did her best to lie to the patient, telling him she had not seen his notes and suggesting he talk to the doctor in the morning. She made him a cup of tea and chatted until he fell asleep. That was in 1954.

More than three decades later, after several periods as a cancer patient herself, the nurse told a conference in London how much remorse she still felt at that deception, and pleaded for more openness from health professionals in their dealings with people suffering from cancer. Enormous courage was needed to put that question into words and patients should be answered truthfully, she said.

When the doctor chairing the conference, on communication problems in cancer, asked how many of the audience would still feel unable to answer that question truthfully, more than half the nurses in the audience put up their hands.

The wisdom of decreeing such questions 'off limits' for nurses trusted with the administration of powerful drugs and round-the-clock care of patients is open to doubt. And to an outside observer it appears to have as much to do with the hospital hierarchies as the needs of the patients.

Traditionally, discussion of diagnosis has been the pre-rogative of doctors, and many are happy for it to remain so, be-lieving they do a reasonably good job of telling patients about their condition, despite the restrictions on their time.

Nurses, on the other hand, know that patients ask again and again about their illness, putting the questions to anyone close at hand who seems sympathetic. The need, they feel, is for a clear record showing what the patient has been told rather than rigid demarcations about who may speak openly and who may not. And so the debate about who should tell what, and when, goes on.

What is not open to doubt is the burden that communication problems often represent for the person with cancer. Personal ac-counts including those of doctors and nurses who have developed cancer show that the sense of loss, isolation and bewilderment can be as hard to bear as any of the disease's physical manifestations; often more so because the emotions are unexpected.

Many people with newly diagnosed cancer look, and often feel, completely normal. But their world has been overturned and may be dominated by uncertainty for months, and sometimes years.

Just when their need for closeness is strongest they may sense a distancing of family. And friends may drop them completely without any explanation, leaving the person with cancer feeling 'written off' in the cruellest way.

For someone coping with initial reactions to the diagnosis of cancer – shock, anger, denial, depression – it can be very hard indeed to be outgoing and to adopt a deliberately assertive attitude.

But it is likely to pay dividends. In many cases partners, children, friends and doctors will be waiting to take their cue from you – about how much you want to know and how the illness is to be approached. So it is beneficial to make it clear how you intend to tackle treatment and the illness itself. Most people dislike uncertainty and don't know how to approach people in sad or difficult situations. Often it will be up to you to make the first move, by inviting them round, asking them to do something for you. The longer the silence the worse their fears are likely to be. It is unfair that someone already feeling at a disadvantage through illness should have to make the approaches. But that is how it often is.

GETTING THE DOCTORS TO TALK TO YOU

Nobody has succeeded in making anyone else immortal, but doctors seem to feel that failure more sharply than most. Trained to think along the lines of treating and curing they feel inadequate when their purposes are frustrated, as they often are with cancer. All too often, they admit, their general feelings of guilt and failure about cancer are transferred to individual patients. Several recent conferences have explored the idea that it is doctors who reinforce the general public's fear of cancer, rather than the people actually coping with the disease.

But at the same time cancer is never good news and it is a doctor who brings it. So doctors are a natural focus for a good deal of anger, however they impart the information. Patients often complain of being given their diagnosis in an abrupt, unfeeling way in a brief consultation which gave no time for explanations or questions. Even when explanations are given it is common for patients to come away having forgotten, or simply not taken in, most of what has been said.

Conditions in most clinics are less than ideal and most people are extremely sensitive to the time pressures. They frequently leave with many questions unasked – worried, but concerned about 'bothering the doctor'. But it is difficult to see how anyone can come to terms with a potentially life-threatening illness without giving the doctor the bother of a few questions.

It is worth reminding yourself of that whenever you feel inhibited about asking for information. Cancer affects so many areas of life that nobody can reasonably expect you to face it virtually mute. The doctor may indeed be busy and a poor communicator, but he or she should either tell you what you want to know or refer you to someone who has the time to do so. Several clinics have specialist nurses whose job it is to explain what the diagnosis will mean in terms of treatment and daily life.

A few practical points. After a couple of hours' wait in outpatients your resolve may be weakened, your questions forgotten and your single urge to get home, or back to work, as quickly as possible. Some people find it helpful to make a list of everything they want to know before setting out for hospital. And taking a partner or companion, now actively encouraged by some hospitals, not only eases the wait but provides moral support and valuable back-up should you forget what the doctor said. One elderly man with lung cancer took both his daughters to all his hospital appointments and they were only once asked to leave while the doctor did an examination. This man felt much more relaxed when someone else was with him who could ask the questions and write down the answers.

Where hospitals operate an appointment system as opposed to block booking (everyone arriving at the same time) you may find you get more time if you take the last appointment. But the realities of the National Health Service mean that doctors and patients have little time to find out about each other and that doctors have to decide, on the basis of a few minutes' consultation, how much, or how little, you want to know.

It is often up to patients to reveal something of themselves and their general approach to life if the doctor is to respond appropriately. The fact that some people do say 'It's up to you, doctor, do whatever you think is best' does not mean that doctors expect unquestioning passivity. It is often up to the patient to show what is required and how much discussion and explanation is expected.

Hilary Baker was 31 when cancer of the tongue was diagnosed. She underwent surgery, followed by radiotherapy, and then, when that did not work, a second operation to remove part of her tongue, which necessitated her having speech therapy.

She feels doctors involved with cancer patients should be more aware of the need for good communication. 'Most people only become patients very occasionally, but doctors meet millions of patients, so the onus should be on them to make the relationship work,' she says.

'When I asked the houseman what would happen if the radiotherapy didn't work he said "you may be run over by a big red bus by then" ... not very helpful, when what you want is information.

'But the consultant was very good and made me feel we were a team, going to beat this thing together. When I asked what would happen if I didn't have treatment he said I could be dead in two or three months. I appreciated that – someone who cared about me being straightforward and honest.'

TALKING TO YOUR PARTNER

Sadly, a diagnosis of cancer can drive couples apart, just when they need each other most. But it can also strengthen partnerships and many couples report improved closeness and understanding as a result of facing the illness together.

This is most likely to happen where partners tackle cancer as a common problem, likely to affect them both deeply, albeit in different ways. There is no quick, straightforward way of facing up to a life-threatening condition. And whether it is one's own life threatened or that of a beloved, any adjustment must be gradual, but is helped by a deliberate concentration on the present, rather than continual worrying about an unknown future.

Peter Morris, a freelance medical journalist, was 38 when he was found to have lung cancer. He had been feeling extremely tired for 18 months and was suffering from sweating attacks at night, but first thought his condition was psychosomatic.

He had an operation to remove the tumour from his lung and was told he had a 30 per cent chance of survival. 'The doctors were wonderful and told me anything I wanted to know. I was always very optimistic. But it was a hard time for my wife, Gloria. As soon as the news leaked out the telephone never stopped ringing.

'It upset her much more than it did me and I think that's often the way. The person with cancer is cosseted in hospital, the centre of attention, but the relatives and friends are worse off.'

Gloria, a teacher, although calm when Peter told her his diagnosis in hospital, suffered quite severe shock afterwards.

'For two or three days I was all right – then I found I couldn't go to work. I was shaking, trembling and exhausted and still can't remember a lot of what happened. My doctor gave me pills to calm me down. When Peter came out of hospital between the diagnosis and the operation we visited friends and I just didn't know what I was saying.'

Sympathetic telephone calls from friends provided a 'horrific' drain on her strength while she was working full-time and then visiting Peter in hospital. 'It was often midnight before I got dinner, so many people rang up and I had to repeat the same thing again and again.'

More than three years on, Peter, formerly a sixty-a-day smoker, feels well, and swims and cycles despite diminished lung function. 'I exercise a lot as a sort of white magic. But I think cancer is largely behind me ... not like the first year when I thought I had a recurrence every time I woke up hot.'

He celebrated the first anniversary of his operation by cycling twelve miles and swimming one mile. Always 'slightly preoccupied' by Peter's health, Gloria likes to make plans year by year rather than looking further into the future.

WHAT CAN YOU SAY TO YOUR CHILDREN?

There is growing agreement among doctors and nurses that children with cancer almost always know the seriousness of their condition and look for opportunities to discuss it with those close to them.

The questions asked vary according to the age of the child, but are best answered as openly as possible by parents; otherwise the child is at risk of losing trust and confidence in those he or she had previously relied on.

Shocked at the diagnosis, parents may decide there should be no discussion of the illness, either with the child, or within the family. But hopes of sparing the child distress in this way are likely to prove unrealistic.

Once the subject of extensive tests, repeated hospital visits and whispered conversations, few children can accept assurances about there being nothing to worry about. But they will pick up the signal that parents are too distressed to talk about the situation and so decide to keep their fears to themselves, whatever the personal cost.

Elaborate attempts at concealment are bound to fail in the face of an illness which may go on for months or years. Few families can convincingly live a lie, day in day out, and attempts to do so will merely increase the child's feeling of isolation and abandonment. Also, the severity of the treatment makes it obvious to the child that the condition must be serious.

Children seek reassurance that they can rely on the continuing support of those close to them in facing the unknown, and have a right to expect it. Doctors report that while 50 per cent of children with cancer will survive to normal adult life, many have psychological handicaps as a result of being denied information about their illness and explanations of treatments. Some doctors insist children of school age be told they have cancer, before they hear a garbled version of their illness in the playground. It is important for children to be given opportunities to discuss possible resentments at side-effects, such as hair loss, and for schools to be alerted to changes in the appearance of a child returning after cancer treatment. In some areas hospital social workers make a point of talking to the relevant class to clear up prejudices about cancer being catching, before a child's return from cancer treatment. Similarly, when it is a parent who has cancer, children will benefit from being kept in the picture and having their questions answered honestly.

*

Andrew Svvennsen was 12 when he came back from the beach unable to walk properly. He had suffered a series of headaches and nosebleeds, which his mother, Averil, a trained nurse, first interpreted as being part of his adjusting to a new secondary school. Then he started vomiting and underwent a complete change of personality, getting angry over trifles. Within a week he was in hospital and a cancerous tumour was diagnosed in the centre of his brain. After an eight-hour exploratory operation surgeons decided that it could not be removed. Andrew spent almost four months in hospital in London, undergoing radiotherapy and chemotherapy. His mother stayed with him all the time, leaving his brother Kai, then 14, and 10-year-old sister Naomi in the care of friends.

'The other children lived a nightmare while we were up at the hospital,' recalls Averil. 'This is a small town and everywhere they went there were people whispering about Andrew and how he was dying. I decided right from the start to be totally truthful. From my nursing days I remember couples playing a sort of cat-and-mouse game, not talking about the illness, when they both knew. I found that upsetting. Having shared life, they were apart, just when they needed to be together.

'I made a pact with myself that if I were ever confronted with cancer there would be no pretending and I never regretted that.'

She told Andrew as much as she could about his condition and the treatments, urging doctors to do the same, and telephoned his brother and sister regularly to report progress.

After coming home Andrew spent two years in a wheel chair before returning, very gradually, to normal life, going back to school for short periods, at first.

Although frustrated at being unable to play tennis and football for so long, and dismayed when he had to make new friends at school after his long absence, Andrew never felt bitter about his illness and believes it increased his understanding of the sick and dependent, as well as deepening his faith in God. It is vitally important, he feels, to maintain your identity and determination, whenever threatened with being treated like a non-person.

'People would ignore me when I was in the wheel chair and whisper to Mum "What's wrong with him?" I used to say "I've got cancer" and stare back,' he recalls. 'In hospital when they whispered at the foot of my bed I used to ask them to speak up and remind them it was my head they were talking about. I got really annoyed when the doctors didn't tell me what was going on.'

Averil, a single parent, found the time after Andrew came out of hospital the most taxing. As well as running the home she had to look after someone still extremely weak. And, inevitably, there were many readjustments to be made within the family. Naomi admits it was hard to lose her place as centre of attention, as the youngest and only girl, and she and Kai resented always being referred to as 'Andrew's brother and sister'. It was hard when well-wishers ignored the strain they had been under.

'We tried very hard to make it equal all round, but it's impossible,' recalls Averil. 'If you've got a child in a wheel chair with no hair he has to get more attention than anyone else.' But the long-term effects on the family were all good. 'We've become much closer and more considerate.'

Although the radiotherapy affected his growth, and concentration is a greater effort than before, Andrew was sitting exams and, four years on, had no recurrence of the cancer. 'I like to be active all the time and keep setting myself new goals. I'm determined to get my six-mile run down to 40 minutes,' he said.

TALKING TO ADOLESCENTS

Teenagers' reactions to cancer in the family, like their reactions to most things, are likely to vary from day to day and can extend to violent resentment and denial.

Some doctors and nurses believe that adolescents are the least equipped to cope with cancer, either in themselves or others. When they are trying to establish their independence they feel affronted by illness in a parent which may involve them having to do more at home. Some actually voice their anger at a mother who develops breast cancer just before their exams. When a brother or sister has cancer there is often resentment among siblings about one child drawing what seems like all the parents' attention.

Situations which cannot be 'settled' seem to be especially disturbing to teenagers and they may find the uncertainty of cancer almost unbearable, even if they do not show it. It is always a good idea to put the school in the picture in case of changes in behaviour or standard of school work.

REALISTIC RELATIONSHIPS

Looked at objectively it is obvious that one person's needs cannot consistently take precedence above those of all others in a group. But cancer often comes as such a shock to partners and families that objectivity goes out the window and everyone determines to concentrate on the person with the disease to the exclusion of their relationships with each other and almost everything else. People often set themselves impossibly high standards of commitment and unflagging care and are surprised at the strain, resentment and sheer exhaustion this engenders. All this is eased if, early on, it is recognized that cancer is stressful for all those involved, not just the person with the disease.

'I WOULDN'T KNOW WHERE TO BEGIN'

Friends and families often ask what they should say to people with cancer and are worried about putting their foot in it, or giving the 'wrong reaction'. There is no formula, but often it is a question of listening and being ready to take your cue from the person concerned, and having confidence in the relationship and what you shared before the diagnosis.

Generally speaking the simpler the approach the better. A simple 'How are you?' or 'How is it going at the hospital?' gives the person an opening to say as much, or as little, as they want to at that time. They may indicate that they are upset and not willing to expand at the moment. In that case it is probably best to let them lead the conversation for the moment, while conveying through your expression and tone that you are open should they wish to talk about their feelings at some later stage.

Rushing in with a torrent of false assurances the moment the person with cancer expresses any distress is to be avoided. That will be taken as a clear sign that you are unable, or unwilling, to share others' suffering. And very likely, you will not be offered another chance.

Where the person concerned has not yet discussed their diagnosis they may 'test the water' with you, saying something like 'I don't seem to be getting any better' or 'It seems to be quite serious'. If you reply 'Nonsense, we'll soon have you back on the cricket field' or 'Of course you're getting better, we all need you' that person will take the hint that their true situation and feelings are out of bounds for discussion. And their sense of rejection can be immense. It is far better to say quietly 'Yes it looks like that' or 'It seems so' and let them take it from there.

While nobody with cancer wants, or expects, their state of health to be the subject of every conversation, they have a right to some acknowledgment that they are coping with a crisis.

Breezing in with boisterous talk of the football scores, the stock exchange or the boss in the belief that this will distract and keep the person in touch with the outside world is a mistake. Often they are, quite naturally, preoccupied with their personal world, which has been suddenly overturned with uncertainty.

Percy Helman, a surgeon who recorded his feelings on developing bowel cancer, described how offensive he found visitors who rushed into the room saying how marvellous he looked when he knew he looked like 'all hell'. After that he felt he could not believe anything they had to say. He most appreciated those who held his hand and quietly admitted that they didn't know what to say.

The fact that people living with cancer often look perfectly normal should not be taken as a reason for never mentioning their treatment, or for not inquiring about their health. However well they respond to treatment and appear to have put cancer behind them it is worth bearing in mind that they have been faced with their own mortality. And very often they feel diminished, and at some disadvantage to those who never have to give their own health a second thought.

We all know how easy it is to feel at a disadvantage when faced with those who are brighter, better looking or evidently more successful than ourselves. But we frequently fail to recognize the vulnerability of those who can no longer take good health, that most basic asset, for granted. It merits some consideration.

This is not to say that people with cancer do not look to family and friends for fun, diversion and stimulus. Far from it. They want relationships to continue as before, but with some consideration of their changed circumstances. Their confidence and ability to take life and health for granted have taken a severe shaking.

DENYING THE TRUTH

Temporary or complete denial is a way of coping with un-pleasant experiences. Many people, especially immediately after diagnosis, appear not to have taken in information about their condition and may deny that cancer has ever been mentioned.

Whether or not people continue to deny their illness depends to some extent on how they have coped with previous crises and with continuing difficulties. But reactions from partners and family also play a part. It is not at all uncommon for both partners to hide their knowledge of the illness from the other, each fearing that the other 'would go to pieces'. Similarly some spouses insist doctors must not let the patient know the true diagnosis. Some doctors will go along with this in some cases, such as that of the elderly patient already coping with severe physical problems. But, faced with a direct question from the patient, no doctor is likely to lie.

While some people do decide that the only way they can cope with a life-threatening illness is to work on, behaving as if nothing has happened, it is questionable whether this really makes things easier in the long run. Denying a problem does not dissolve the difficulty but blocks off potential support from others. Acting normally, when everything is palpably far from normal, puts an immense strain on families. Some sharing of the fears and upset can bring great relief. And without it individuals can easily believe that they are the only ones to find the situation so worrying. Each feels under a strong obligation to 'put a good face on it' for the sake of the others.

HOW LONG WILL IT BE, DOCTOR?

Some doctors maintain that patients never ask this. Others say this question is almost inevitable, from relatives if not from the person with cancer, especially from those looking after someone who is evidently very sick.

Most doctors are unhappy about giving exact answers, and for several reasons. How the cancer will develop and respond to treatment is extremely difficult to predict, and some women with breast cancer die within two years, for example, while others survive for a normal lifespan. Some forms of the disease, such as lung cancer, are more predictable than others. But with any type of cancer, a proportion of people will survive to be totally cured. And doctors are unhappy about making predictions when, medically, they know they are on shaky ground.

But there is also a deeper reason. Doctors are human, however they may sometimes appear. And faced with acute distress and uncertainty we all want to offer reassurance. Medics more so than most; that is why they went into the job in the first place. They know, of course, that many cancers will not prove curable and that many of their patients will, at some time, die from their condition. But they do not want to take away the individual's hope, or will to live. And once they've given any sort of 'time-limit' there's a risk that they'll do just that. Given two months to live, or whatever, some people will go away and literally wait for death. And most doctors have seen this phenomenon at work.

One regular visitor to the Bristol Cancer Help Centre tells how she was once given two months to live and started crossing off the days on a calendar. Two weeks before her allotted span was up she realized that she was behaving ridiculously and that she could control the quality of her life, if not prolong it. So she stopped waiting for death and started to concentrate on living, and has outlived the original prediction by several years.

So apart from feeling unable, on professional grounds, to answer the 'how-long' question, doctors also wonder how much benefit or relief an uncertain answer will prove to people with cancer and their families. Relatives who make plans on the basis of a doctor's prediction often become extremely angry when the disease doesn't behave as expected and they have to cancel a holiday or whatever. This may seem base, but it's true.

All this may seem like so much eyewash if you are the person facing the doctor and asking the question. But when doctors hesitate, and say they do not know, they are not simply stalling out of self-protection.

Cancer *is* unpredictable and anyone affected by it must somehow come to terms with that uncertainty. This is one of the most demanding aspects of the illness. But all of us, at all stages in life, want to know how long we will be asked to bear difficulties and unhappiness. So you should ask about the range of probabilities and persist if you feel you are being palmed off. Always remember it is not the doctor who has cancer, and if more information will help you to cope then keep on until you get it. It is entirely natural to ask the doctor 'How long?' But the answer may not always bring the relief you are looking for.

When people with cancer say 'Is it fatal?' or 'How long have I got?', far from wanting one-line answers they are often after an explanation of what they can expect in terms of their own capabilities and autonomy and whether they will become dependent. However many patients they see, doctors rarely become mind-readers. You must indicate the areas of your main concern when asking such questions. 'I want to put my affairs in order and plan for the family' is more likely to produce helpful opinion than 'How long have I got?'

If you are worried about possible pain, or incontinence, dependence or the strain on your partner, say so. Often doctors are waiting to take their cue from you about the sort of information and support you want.

TALKING TO FRIENDS

Friends can become extremely precious to those coping with cancer – a link with the normal world away from hospitals and worried relatives. It can be a great relief for someone in a highly charged atmosphere to have the normal distractions of visiting a friend, or going out to lunch.

Yet sometimes people draw away when they hear someone has cancer. They feel frightened and believe they should do something superhuman to help. Rather than risk failure or distress they distance themselves completely. From the point of view of the person with cancer, nothing could be further from the truth. They do not require spectacular support, but do want to hang on to normal life as much as possible. So many assumptions and expectations have been overturned that fixed points, such as friendship and regular social occasions, acquire extra significance. Never assume that in some mysterious way the person with cancer will be too 'busy' for the weekly lunch or the drink after work; that can all too easily be interpreted as rejection.

If possible choose a quiet moment to tell friends about the

diagnosis when neither of you is rushed or surrounded by other people. Avoid ringing them at work when they are very unlikely to be able to talk freely or to give you the concentration they would like. And be prepared for negative reactions. Some people will simply be unable to give the understanding you warrant or to put aside their own preoccupations. Some people find it easy to reorder their priorities, while others take time to absorb stressful situations and may say something harsh or dismissive-sounding without really meaning it. Others, sadly, are always too busy to put themselves out to ease the lot of others. The smoothest way is never to expect anything from these people and never to count on them, however much you feel you deserve their loyalty. Sadly, some people simply cannot bear others' misfortunes and will often lose very little time in showing it. Most people with cancer report at least one relative or friend who never got in contact again after hearing the diagnosis. The only way to minimize the hurt of such reactions is to look on them as expressions of inadequacy rather than considered rejections. Often they are based on the person's own fears of illness and uncertainty and should not be taken too personally.

Whether or not you decide to try again to contact the person in a few months' time depends how much the relationship means to you. You may decide it is not worth it.

*

Comedy actor Felix Bowness, Fred Quilley in the television series *Hi-de-Hi*, was in a summer season in Bognor when he discovered a speck of blood coming from a small spot on his cheek. It was found to be a rodent ulcer, a type of skin cancer.

He underwent four operations, over several years, to have it removed, as well as radiotherapy, but only ever missed one performance. Three years ago he was told he was cured and is now an active fund-raiser for his local radiotherapy unit.

'When I first heard I was terrified. I thought "Oh God, an actor with cancer of the face," and I didn't tell the cast because I was afraid they would keep away from me.

'But when they did find out we joked about it and they gave me a lot of support. Now I am completely open about having had cancer. And if I had to go back for more treatment it wouldn't worry me.'

Chapter Four

MAKING DECISIONS

'The death certificate has not been signed the day the diagnosis is made. There is always some treatment possible.' (Professor Tim McElwain, Royal Marsden Hospital, London)

As if the discovery of cancer were not shattering enough, many people are expected to make important decisions about treatment with the dreaded words still ringing in their ears. Before they have had time to take in what is wrong with them they are being offered major surgery, radiotherapy, chemotherapy – options they may have heard of but know little about.

There is no doubt that once cancer is diagnosed it is important to begin treatment as soon as possible. The chances of successfully treating a small tumour are greater than with a large one. But many tumours will have taken months or even years to reach the hundreds of millions of cells which can be picked up in modern diagnostic tests. So will a few days' delay in deciding on treatment make any difference?

The answer has to be 'no' for the vast majority of people; in fact, many specialist cancer doctors do encourage people to go home and think about things after they are first told that they have cancer. They should talk about the possible treatments with their friends and relatives, and go back to their doctor to discuss anything which worries them. And only when they are sure that they understand what are the options for treatment, what they are aiming to do and how they will be carried out should they decide what to do.

There are exceptions: acute leukaemia, certain types of testicular cancer which can double in size in a few days, a tumour pressing on the spinal cord which needs immediate action to avoid permanent paralysis. But these are rare.

This is not to encourage delays of weeks or months, but it does mean that there is rarely a need for the kind of rushed decisions still forced on many people newly diagnosed with cancer in out-patients' clinics. Some people would rather leave the decisions to their doctors. Every day, people ask their doctors what they would do in their position. It is a good question and generally gets an honest answer. There is nothing wrong with acting unquestioningly on the advice of your doctor if that is the way which enables *you* to deal best with a difficult situation.

But if that is not your way and you want to make the decisions you will need certain basic information. Your doctor will outline the options for treatment, but perhaps the most important question to ask is 'What are you trying to do?'

THE AIMS OF TREATMENT

Don't be fobbed off with an answer like 'We're trying to make you better': surely that's common sense! What you need to know is whether the doctor is proposing treatment which stands a good chance of actually curing your illness or whether he is aiming to prolong your life and relieve your symptoms. 'Prolong' is a very open-ended word and it can mean weeks, months or years. So you should not be disheartened if your doctor tells you that, in all honesty, he does not believe that the treatment will cure your cancer. It can still mean that you will have several extra years which it is unlikely that you would have without treatment.

Quite rightly, doctors are careful about using the word 'cure' in relation to cancer. There is a similar feeling about using the word with regard to alcoholism. A relapse is possible at any time. But people with cancer should not feel that there is always a sword hanging over their head about to strike them down. In general, the more time that passes without a recurrence after you have had treatment the less likely it becomes that your cancer will return. The risk of recurrence varies widely between different types of cancer, but your chances of cure will also depend on the size of your tumour and how far it had spread when it was treated. If you have a fast-growing tumour you will know quite quickly whether there is a good chance that you have been cured because there is no early recurrence. But if you have a slower growing tumour you may have to wait some years before you know whether there is a good chance that you are in the clear. Getting a recurrence does not always mean that you cannot be cured. There is no reason why further treatment should not get rid of the cancer for good. It simply means that you will have to wait longer to find out if you are clear.

MEASURING THE SUCCESS OF TREATMENT

To make some sense of all this, doctors compare treatments on the basis of groups of people surviving five and then ten years after their cancer is treated. Such figures vary enormously for different types of cancer. Thus around 60 per cent of middle-aged women can expect to survive five years after being treated for breast cancer compared to less than 10 per cent of middle-aged people with lung cancer.

Statistics can imply a good or bad chance of cure, but doctors do not like using the word even when the outcome looks extremely good. Take skin cancer, for example. With the exception of melanoma, over 95 per cent of young people with skin tumours survive five years after treatment. That still means that around five per cent don't. Anyone with skin cancer can be told that their chances of cure are exceedingly good, though this will depend on the type of tumour they have, but there can still be no guarantees.

This does not mean that we cannot be told the aims of treatment. Where the tumour is diagnosed early doctors will be going for a cure and in some tumours good cure rates are possible even when the tumour is well advanced. But in certain solid tumours, such as lung and bowel cancers, the chances of cure are less good, especially when the tumours have spread. In these cases treatment may be geared towards prolonging life or making people feel well enough to live relatively normal lives.

The extra time which treatment can buy varies enormously, from a few months with chemotherapy for small-cell lung tumours to several years with hormone treatment for advanced breast cancer.

WEIGHING THE BENEFITS OF TREATMENT AGAINST THE RISKS

Treatment geared towards prolonging life rather than cure is called palliative; it does not simply mean the beginning of the end, it can mean several years of active life. The reason it is important to know whether the doctor is attempting potentially curative or palliative treatment is that this will enable you to weigh up the benefits of treatment against the side-effects.

All drugs have side-effects, none more so than those used to treat cancer. Much can be done to alleviate the unpleasant effects of both radiotherapy and chemotherapy but anyone starting such a course of treatment should be satisfied of the advantages.

If there is a good chance of cure or at least of several extra years of enjoyable life then someone with cancer will probably be prepared to put up with the side-effects of treatment – whether that is some kind of disfigurement resulting from surgery, debilitation following radiotherapy or side-effects from drugs. If, however, the treatment is to provide only a few extra months then it may be preferable to refuse treatment and spend the last weeks or months free of the physical and psychological side-effects of treatment. Also in the equation must be the effect of treatment on the quality of life. In some cases the disease can be expected to take a course which will cause far more discomfort than the side-effects of treatment.

There are no easy answers and people vary both in the intensity of side-effects they experience and in how they view the balance between extra life and side-effects. We all cling to life and, given the choice, we may be prepared to put up with unpleasant side-effects for even a few extra months of life. We may prefer to remain unaware of the poor chances of success of treatment and accept whatever is on offer. Or we may be determined that we will be in that small percentage of people who do live for more than a year with even the most lethal forms of cancer.

WHAT ARE THE OPTIONS?

At the very least there are two options after cancer is diagnosed: treatment or no treatment. Most people do choose to have some treatment, but doctors do not simply wash their hands of those who don't. If they wish, people can continue to have regular appointments to see how their cancer is progressing. This gives doctors a chance to recommend ways of making life more comfortable and of course giving people a chance to change their mind about treatment.

TUMOURS IN ONLY ONE AREA

When a tumour is small, easily accessible and limited to one specific area the simplest and most effective way of treating it is to remove it surgically. This can be done with bowel tumours, tumours of skin and bone, breast tumours and some lung cancers.

Sometimes the tumour may have lodged deep in a vital organ such as the brain or liver and it is impossible to operate because of the damage which would be done to the surrounding tissue. Or, quite simply, it has been found that other forms of treatment, such as radiotherapy or chemotherapy, are more effective. For example, radiotherapy is highly effective in Hodgkin's disease – a cancer of the immune system. And chemotherapy is excellent in treating leukaemia.

If there are no signs that a tumour has spread when removed surgically then no further treatment may be needed. But in some cases doctors may recommend some more treatment to mop up any tumour cells which may have escaped the surgeon. This may be radiotherapy or chemotherapy. Sometimes one or other of these techniques may be recommended before surgery. This is in order to shrink the tumour and make it easier for the surgeon to get rid of it.

TUMOURS WHICH HAVE SPREAD

Once a tumour has spread to other parts of the body it is less likely that surgery or radiotherapy will be able to help. Of course, there are exceptions, and if a tumour has spread to only one or two other places, affecting relatively small areas, it may be possible to remove the new tumours surgically or with radiotherapy.

Where this is not possible, doctors turn to chemotherapy. Drugs put into the bloodstream can reach the parts which surgery and radiotherapy cannot reach. There is a risk that they will also attack healthy cells but, in general, drugs used in chemotherapy prefer tumour to normal cells, and new methods of targeting these drugs aim to make them even more specific in the way they attack cancer cells.

Like radiotherapy, chemotherapy is also used to mop up any rogue cancer cells which may have escaped the surgeon. There may be obvious signs that the tumour has spread, or just a suspicion, based on experience, that the tumour may already be on its way elsewhere.

WHAT DO YOU NEED TO KNOW ABOUT SURGERY?

It is remarkable how little some of us know about what is going to happen when we enter the operating theatre. Anyone down for surgery has to sign a consent form or, if they are too ill to do so, a close relative must sign. How often do they wonder what they are letting themselves in for as they sign on the dotted line!

There are three main reasons for surgery in cancer:
1. An exploratory operation to look for cancer and to take samples of tissue for examination under a microscope (biopsy).
2. To remove the tumour in an effort to cure the cancer.
3. To remove part or all of the tumour in order to reduce discomfort or for some other palliative reason.

BIOPSIES

Widespread use of body scanners and ultrasound machines has helped reduce the need for so-called 'exploratory' operations. Where once they would have had to open up the body to have a look and see what was wrong, doctors can now use X-rays or sound waves to pick up many tumours. But while these machines can tell them that there is a growth, they are unable to determine whether it is benign or malignant. Doctors need to be able to get hold of a piece of the growth and look at its cells under the microscope.

In some cases it is possible to do this without a full-scale operation. Thousands of women each year have cervical smears. A small sample of cells is taken from the neck of the womb by passing a swab over the lining of the cervical canal. Done carefully, the sample is taken painlessly in seconds without the need for any anaesthetic. Samples of cells can be taken from superficial lumps in other areas of the body with only a local anaesthetic; cells from simple skin lumps, for example.

Samples of cells can even be taken from passages deep in the body without the need for a full operation. Lumps in the tubes to the lungs can be examined by passing a tube (bronchoscope) down through the mouth and into the 'bronchi' – the passages which take air to the lungs. The tube contains fine glass fibres which relay light and enable the doctor to see the lump through an eyepiece. A similar machine (endoscope) can be used to look down into the stomach and upper intestine from the mouth, or up into the lower part of the intestine via the rectum (colonoscope). Once the doctor has spotted the lump it is possible to pass a probe down the tube into it and remove a sample of cells. These can then be taken to the laboratory, stained with chemicals and examined under the microscope.

Sometimes it is not possible to take a sample in this way and the only option is to perform a small operation and remove part of the lump. This is generally when the lump is not in a hollow tube but in the tissue itself, such as the breast or kidney, for example. This then has to be done under general anaesthetic.

SURGERY WHICH AIMS TO CURE

When a tumour is clearly defined and quite small it is possible to remove it surgically with a good prospect of 'cure'. Since laboratory examination of biopsy material can now be carried out very quickly, surgeons frequently like to do both the biopsy and removal of the tumour, if this is what it proves to be, at the same operation. Unfortunately, removing the tumour frequently means that the surrounding tissue must go as well because of the risk that the tumour has spread into it.

Before going into the operating theatre it is very important to find out exactly what the doctor has in mind. Is he or she simply going to take a sample of cells and then send you back to the ward to await the results? Or will the operation to remove any cancer which is found go ahead straightaway? Sometimes it is entirely sensible to go ahead with the major operation – both to avoid the small risks of a second general anaesthetic and to get rid of the tumour as quickly as possible. But in some cases it may be better to have a breathing space, time to reconsider the options and to come to terms with the implications.

Rarely is this more true than in the case of breast cancer. Women are still wheeled into the operating theatre without knowing whether or not they will lose a breast and wake up to discover what the surgeon has decided on their behalf. There is no reason why you should not decide to leave it to the surgeon's judgement on what to do when he gets the biopsy results; the important thing is that *you* decided.

With something like breast cancer it is important to find out your surgeon's practice concerning removal of lumps. There is good evidence that in many cases removal of the lump itself, generally accompanied by radiotherapy and sometimes chemotherapy, is just as effective as removal of the whole breast. Yet a survey published in 1985 showed that the majority of British surgeons are continuing to perform mastectomies in spite of evidence showing that many may not be necessary. So it is important to find out the approach of your own particular surgeon:

- In what situation would he do a mastectomy and when would he do a lumpectomy?
- What additional treatment would he recommend – radiotherapy/chemotherapy/hormones?

Similar sorts of questions can be asked with other types of cancer.

Some doctors are not keen to answer this sort of 'what if' question. They don't want to raise hopes by suggesting that it may be possible to do a conservative operation before they have been able to see exactly what they are dealing with. Equally they don't want to depress you by telling you what may be necessary if things don't look so good when they open you up – after all, it may never happen. Such reservations are understandable, but you have a right to know what you are letting yourself in for. You may not choose to exercise that right. But make sure you have all the information you want before you go into the operating theatre.

SURGERY TO RELIEVE SYMPTOMS

Many cancer operations are performed not to get rid of all the tumour but to relieve discomfort or remove cancerous tissue which is threatening vital organs. Advanced tumours in the intestines may impair or completely block the passage of food and waste products with potentially lethal consequences. Likewise, diseased tissue which is pressing on blood vessels may prevent proper blood-flow to healthy tissues causing them to become diseased or die. Nerves pinched between cancerous and healthy tissue can become very painful. Palliative operations may be carried out at any time after cancer is diagnosed. The object may be to prevent symptoms before they occur or to relieve them once they have started.

HOW RADIOTHERAPY IS GIVEN

Many people with cancer will be given radiotherapy at some point in their treatment. The most commonly used forms of radiation are X-rays and gamma rays. They are just two of the many waves, rays and particles to which we are exposed in very small amounts in the atmosphere. For the purposes of radiotherapy, X-rays and gamma rays have the same properties and can be used interchangeably, but X-rays can be produced electrically while gamma rays must come from a radioactive source, most commonly cobalt. The equipment looks much the same but the radiocobalt unit which gives off gamma rays is rather smaller and less powerful than the linear accelerator which produces X-rays.

Most of us over the age of 20 think of X-rays in terms of the mobile units which trundled from town to town in the 1950s and 1960s to take pictures of our lungs and ensure that there were no signs of tuberculosis. But the dose of radiation each of us receives from an ordinary chest X-ray is only a fraction of that achieved by either the radiocobalt unit or the linear accelerator. In fact, a course of radiation is around five million times more powerful than the average diagnostic X-ray. Taken out of context, figures like that sound rather frightening, but remember that the object is to destroy a tumour of perhaps billions of cells or more, and even more important than the power of the radiation is the way it is adapted to strike at the diseased rather than the healthy tissue.

Before a course begins, ordinary diagnostic X-rays are taken to pin-point precisely the area of tissue to be treated. It is not just a case of marking on the skin the point at which the rays will enter the body; those performing the treatment must know exactly how far the rays must penetrate. And what of the tissues in between? Courses are plotted so that no healthy tissue gets more than a small dose of radiation. This is done by aiming the rays from different directions. It is a bit like moving troops to a battleground. If you send them all along the same route there will be such a traffic jam that it will take months to get them in position and the weight of equipment will probably destroy the road! But if you break the troops down into groups and have them converge on the battleground from all directions they will get there more quickly and do less damage to the roads. So it is with radiotherapy; the total dose arriving at the tumour is the same but the tissues *en route* receive less damage if the rays are broken down and sent in from several different directions.

Once the courses are plotted the radiotherapy is generally given over a period of three to six weeks, either daily or two or three times a week. Each treatment can last only a few seconds up to several minutes, depending on the individual and how treatment has been planned.

HOW LONG DOES IT TAKE TO WORK?

Tumours vary enormously in how they respond to radiotherapy. Sensitive cancer cells are less able than normal cells to repair the damage caused to them by gamma or X-rays. Just how quickly the effects of radiotherapy can be seen depends on what happens inside each cell attacked by the rays. Sometimes the damage to the genetic material, the DNA, is so great that the cell dies within a few hours. Alternatively, the cell may continue normally until it is time to divide, at which point the damaged DNA is unable to go ahead with the normal process of replication. As we have already seen, cancer cells in general tend to divide more quickly than healthy cells, so this second effect of the radiotherapy may happen within a few days of treatment. Those cells with longer life cycles live on for a while but, because they are sterile, they slowly degenerate and die. This can take several months, which is why the full benefits of a course of radiotherapy may take some time to show themselves.

Increasingly, gamma rays are being used to treat small, localized tumours by inserting tiny rods or wires of radioactive material into the cancer site instead of using the large radiocobalt units as external sources of radiation. These wires release their radioactivity over a period of days or weeks and are then removed. The technique has proved particularly useful in mouth, breast and uterine cancers.

DOES RADIOTHERAPY HURT?

Courses of radiotherapy are carefully planned so that they cause as little damage as possible to healthy tissue. The skin over the treated area may become red and sore – a little like sunburn. Protective guards may well be put over certain parts of your body to prevent the treatment damaging healthy tissue. (Since frequent, unnecessary exposure to X-rays is dangerous for healthy people, those giving you radiotherapy will stand behind protective shields or in a separate room while you are having treatment.)

Because radiotherapy is geared to the fast-dividing cancer cells it also affects healthy cells which multiply quickly. So blood cells and cells in the mouth and intestine are most frequently damaged by radiotherapy. This leads to some of the most common side-effects – tiredness, mouth ulcers, loss of appetite and nausea; and ways of minimizing or alleviating side-effects are dealt with in the next chapter.

WHAT IS CHEMOTHERAPY?

The word chemotherapy has a mystique it does not deserve because all that it means is 'treatment with medicines'. The medicines which constitute 'chemotherapy' are more toxic than other drugs in common use and have far more serious side-effects. They are, after all, designed to kill cancer cells; it is fortunate that, on the whole, they are far less good at killing most normal healthy cells. (Anti-cancer drugs are frequently referred to as cytotoxic – literally, toxic to cells.)

There are four main groups of anti-cancer drugs: alkylating agents, antibiotics, antimetabolites and mitotic inhibitors.

Alkylating agents are the largest group and they work by attacking the genetic material or DNA which is vital for all functions of cells including growth. By reacting with the DNA of tumour cells these drugs prevent them from dividing and getting bigger. The most commonly used drugs in this group are nitrogen mustard, cyclophosphamide and melphalan.

It probably seems odd that **antibiotics** are used to treat cancer, but these are not the antibiotics such as penicillin which are used to combat common infections. Instead these are antibiotics which are produced by bacteria but have only a weak effect against infections. What they can do, however, is to poison tumour cells. Doxorubicin (adriamycin) is probably the best known drug in this group.

Antimetabolites interfere with the manufacture of DNA of tumour cells. Methotrexate, 6-mercaptopurine (6-MP) and 5-fluorouracil(5-FU) fall into this category.

The **mitotic inhibitors** prevent cells from dividing by acting at a rather later stage. The family of chemicals most commonly used for this purpose was taken originally from a form of periwinkle, and vincristine and vinblastine are the best known of this group.

WHICH DRUG WILL I BE GIVEN?

As cancer therapy has developed, doctors have learned which tumours respond best to the different cytotoxic drugs on offer. In general, common solid tumours such as those of the lung and bowel respond less well than cancers of the blood (leukaemias) and lymph nodes (lymphomas). But there are notable exceptions. The platinum-based drugs – cisplatin and more recently carboplatin – have revolutionized the treatment of testicular cancer. But in many cases, chemotherapy remains a palliative rather than a curative form of treatment. Because the drugs work in different ways they are often given in combinations to maximize the attack on the tumour and minimize side-effects. Three, four or five drugs are often given together.

All anti-cancer drugs have side-effects, some more serious than others. Although the drugs are most likely to kill tumour cells they also affect cells which, like tumour cells, reproduce very quickly. In particular this means cells in the bone marrow, the gut and the mouth and it is these parts of the body which are most likely to suffer side-effects.

The bone marrow is the place where blood cells are produced, so chemotherapy can affect supplies of red and white blood cells. Red cells are responsible for transporting oxygen around the body and so a deficiency can make people feel tired and unable to do all the things they would normally be able to do. By killing white cells in the bone marrow, the anti-cancer drugs reduce the body's resistance to infections. So anyone who is being given such treatment will have regular blood tests to check that the immune cells recover sufficiently between treatments to avoid serious infections.

It is the effect of anti-cancer drugs on the platelet cells of the blood which tends to cause bleeding and bruising. The platelets are the cells which help to form scabs on the skin if you scratch or injure yourself. If they are not working properly even the smallest knock or wound can cause a bruise or bleeding.

Sickness is one of the most common side-effects of virtually all anti-cancer drugs. The severity varies according to the person being treated and the particular drug being used. Generally, the sickness starts within a few hours of treatment; nausea may last for a few days. Just how long the problems last depends to some extent on how the drug is given.

The majority of drugs are given directly into a vein. This may be as a simple injection taking a few minutes, or as a drip which allows the drug to slowly get into the blood over a period of about an hour or more. Some drugs, however, can be taken by mouth as capsules or tablets. The drugs which can be taken by mouth tend to be prescribed daily for a course of treatment lasting perhaps one or two weeks, while those drugs which are given by injection or drip tend to be given in a course once every three or four weeks for several months. Just how long treatment is given tends to depend on the individual's response. If the tumour starts to shrink it may be sensible to continue with treatment to see how small it can get. If it responds less well then some other drug may be tried to get a better response. In contrast, for some tumours, a large 'one-off' dose may be given to try to get rid of the cancer once and for all.

People who will need regular intravenous drips of anti-cancer drugs for many months are often fitted with a permanent tube under their skin, called a catheter. There are various types, but in each case a tube is inserted into a vein, generally in the chest. This remains in place and the end which pokes through the skin is plugged until an injection of drugs is required.

In addition to sickness, many drugs get into the cells of the scalp and make the hair fall out. Again, people vary, and so do the drugs. But cyclophosphamide, adriamycin, and vincristine all cause some or all of the hair to fall out.

Many people experience a loss of appetite during chemo-therapy and they frequently suffer from mouth ulcers. Methods of reducing or coping with all these problems are dealt with in the next chapter.

AM I GETTING THE LATEST TREATMENT?

It is quite natural that people embarking on a course of chemotherapy want the latest and most effective treatment. Reports of miracle cancer cures are bound to leave people wondering whether they are getting what is best. Many such reports are premature; witness the disappointment over interferon. Heralded as the breakthrough we had all been waiting for, interferon is only now, five years on, finding its true niche for certain, unfortunately rather rare, types of cancer.

In recent years there have been few major additions to the anti-cancer drug market and none has been dramatically new or revolutionary in its effectiveness. In each case the newer drug has very little difference in effectiveness over the original drug. Slightly more people may respond for slightly longer periods of time. Often, the only obvious advantage is fewer side-effects. This is not to be ignored. The side-effects associated with anti-cancer drugs are very unpleasant and anything which can help reduce them is to be encouraged. Unfortunately, the most significant difference between the new and older drugs is the cost and doctors trying to balance their dwindling drug budgets must often decide whether paying more for newer drugs is justified by fewer side-effects.

GETTING INVOLVED IN DRUG TRIALS

Dozens of new anti-cancer drugs are currently being put through their paces in clinical trials all over the country. Testing these drugs on people with cancer is the only way of finding out whether they have advantages over present therapy. But no one should be included in one of these trials without their permission. If you are asked to take part in tests on a new anti-cancer drug it is important to find out exactly what it is all about:

- What is the new drug being tested?
- Why are you being offered it?
- What evidence is there that it is as good or better than current treatment?
- What side-effects is it expected to have and are these less or greater than those of other established treatment?
- What kind of extra monitoring of how you respond to the drug is planned?
- How easy is it for you to transfer to other treatment if you do not respond well to the new drug?

All plans for trials of new drugs, including anti-cancer drugs, are supposed to be vetted by committees within the hospital to see that they are ethical. There is some debate about whether this always occurs and how strict the procedures are. There are probably very good reasons why you are being asked to take part in a trial of a new drug; without such trials no new drugs would get onto the market. Just be sure that you are happy with the information that you are given about the drug and that getting involved in the trial is in your own best interests as well as those of people with cancer in the future.

WHERE DO HORMONES FIT IN?

As scientists learn more about what makes a cell become cancerous they are also changing their ideas about treatment. Instead of the blunderbuss 'hit it as hard as you can' approach they are moving towards treatment which will alter the underlying mechanisms which go wrong in cancer. For some years they have been aware that some cancers, such as tumours of the breast and prostate, are under some kind of hormonal control.

In the case of breast cancer the main hormones are oestrogens. These are produced by the ovaries from puberty onwards and, amongst other things, are responsible for breast development. It has been shown that some women with breast cancer are especially sensitive to oestrogen and this may have caused cells in their breast to continue multiplying and to get out of control, resulting in the formation of the tumour. Since it is the ovaries that produce oestrogen it has been common practice to remove them in women with recurrent breast tumours which seem to be triggered by oestrogen. Clearly, removing the ovaries is a drastic step for any woman, especially one who has already given up part of her breast. So doctors have sought other ways of blocking the activity of the oestrogen.

A number of drugs have been tested and, at present, the most promising drug is tamoxifen. This has been used to treat advanced breast disease for some years and it is only relatively recently that its value has been recognized for many more women with breast cancer.

A number of clinical trials are underway to identify exactly which women will benefit most. Should it be given to all women who are oestrogen-sensitive after their initial surgery for breast cancer or only if there is a recurrence? Or will the benefits of tamoxifen prove so clear-cut that it should be used actually to prevent breast cancer in women who are at high risk of getting the disease?

It is very important that studies show conclusively how

important tamoxifen is in the treatment and prevention of breast cancer. The cost of giving tamoxifen to large numbers of women at risk of breast cancer would be formidable. And tamoxifen, while having far fewer side-effects than other anti-cancer drugs, is not without its drawbacks.

In their efforts to get ever closer to the source of cancer, scientists are investigating an alternative way of blocking oestrogen, further back in its production pathway. This research will also have important implications for treatment of prostate cancer since this too is under some hormonal influence.

All men get some enlargement of the prostate as they get older, but only a minority develop cancer. The prostate is responsible for producing semen and its development is under the control of androgen from the testes. Current treatment of prostate cancer involves surgery or radiotherapy. If the tumour has spread this is generally accompanied by removal of the testes or the taking of female hormones to combat the production of androgen. Like removal of the ovaries in women with breast cancer, these are drastic measures. A new drug aims to avoid the need for removal of sex organs or administration of hormones to people with breast or prostate cancer by blocking a substance produced in the brain which triggers, via separate pathways, production of androgen in men and of oestrogen in women.

No one knows just how important hormone therapy is going to be in the treatment of cancer or in prevention. Only certain tumours have been shown to come under some hormonal control and, although drugs which block hormones appear to have fewer side-effects than other chemotherapy, they are not entirely free of problems. Like all drugs it will be necessary to show that the benefits of treatment outweigh both the short- and the long-term risks. Hormone therapy does not cure cancer but it does seem to be a useful palliative measure, prolonging and improving the quality of life.

HOW TO GET A SECOND OPINION

Medicine, like most things, is subject to fashion, and the treatment of cancer is no exception. With most cancers there is general agreement as to whether a tumour will be treated most effectively by surgery, radiotherapy or drugs. Most disagreement lies in how those treatments should be carried out. Surgeons have their own preferences in types of operations, and doctors vary in the drugs they use or the doses of radiotherapy they give. Much of the time the differences are small and have little impact on survival.

There are times, however, when you may feel unhappy with the advice you are given about treatment. We have already mentioned how many surgeons still perform a mastectomy for breast cancer when there is good evidence that in many cases a lumpectomy, thus saving the breast, is just as effective. If you are unhappy you can get a second opinion from another doctor.

Under normal circumstances, your general practitioner (GP) will refer you to your local hospital for tests if there is a possibility that you could have a tumour. If cancer is confirmed then the doctors at that same hospital will normally take charge of your treatment. If you have an unusual form of cancer you may be referred to a specialist cancer centre and in some parts of the country people are routinely passed on to the care of doctors who do nothing else but look after people with cancer. But, on the whole, people with cancer are treated by general physicians or surgeons who may have a special interest in a particular part of the body but treat a range of different conditions as well as cancer.

If there is some doubt about the best treatment for you, your doctor at the hospital may bring in a colleague for a second opinion. Or you can ask for a second opinion. Let's face it, this may not go down too well! If you are lucky your doctor will understand your concern and ask one of his colleagues to see you. (If they work together, they may of course hold similar opinions on treatment – and don't forget that that opinion could be right!)

But the doctor treating you at hospital may simply turn down your request for a second opinion; there is no legal obligation for him to call someone else in. Your next option is to go back to your GP and ask to be referred either to a different doctor at the same hospital or to an entirely different hospital. Again, there is no legal obligation on your GP to do this and it may take some pressure from you to get a response. Your appearance daily in the surgery may help!

Hopefully, it will not be a battle of wills and your GP will refer you for a second opinion. If the second doctor gives the same advice then you will have to decide whether or not to take it. It is not unheard of to get a third opinion; this will depend on your relationship with your GP and you should bear in mind the time it could take for new appointments to be made.

What happens if the second doctor recommends something totally different from the first? You will have to be prepared for this as it will probably then be up to you to decide whose advice to take. Your GP may be able to help in interpreting the various options but, having asked for two opinions, the final decision will be yours.

ISN'T THERE ANYTHING ELSE I CAN DO?

This is a question which people ask at all stages of their illness. It may come before any treatment has begun or much later when you've been through the full range of treatment which modern orthodox medicine has to offer. It isn't just a question which people ask when they are feeling ill; some people who have responded well to treatment ask whether there isn't something they can do to prevent the cancer from coming back.

Giving up smoking and eating more fibre and less refined food in your diet can improve general health and help prevent a new cancer developing but they won't stop an old tumour from coming back. The most you can do to prevent a recurrence is to have regular check-ups to catch the earliest signs of any return so that treatment can start.

If you stray outside orthodox medicine there are alternatives. Complementary practitioners believe that cancer, like other diseases, should not be treated on a purely physical basis. Instead, there should be a 'whole body' approach with treatment for mind, body and spirit. There is some evidence that the way someone reacts emotionally to their cancer can affect the outcome. For years, doctors and nurses have noticed that people with a positive approach to all sorts of illnesses seem to do better than those who appear to give up and go away to die. There are no obvious scientific reasons for this, though it has been suggested that positive mental thoughts may somehow stimulate the immune system to beat the illness. It is part of common folklore that people who are depressed seem to be a constant prey to coughs and colds and other minor infections while those who take a much more positive approach to life seem to sail through winter and summer alike without so much as a sniffle.

Complementary therapists believe that particularly in a disease as serious as cancer it is vital to take a positive mental as well as physical approach. Counsellors and therapists attempt to help people with cancer identify emotions and feelings which may have triggered their illness or be working against their recovery. Once identified, they try to modify these negative emotions and make them work for you rather than against you.

Many so called 'alternative' therapists believe that nutrition also has a strong role to play both in preventing and in recovery from cancer. They don't simply advocate 'eat more fibre'; they believe that only fresh food – mainly raw fruit and vegetables with little or no meat or dairy products – can generate the kind of energy which they believe is crucial in the fight against cancer. Such diets are quite complex. Without any meat, you can lose vital proteins which the body simply cannot make up. So various types of bean and cereal are substituted for the missing meat in order to make up the protein content of the diet. Large amounts of enzymes, vitamin and mineral supplements, tailored to individual needs, also form an important part of such diets. And claims are made that these can boost the immune system, destroy cancer cells and flush out toxins. There is no scientific evidence supporting such claims and there are few orthodox doctors who will go along with such ideas. In general they believe that an average, balanced diet of meat and vegetables should contain all the vitamins and minerals necessary for good health and that mega doses of vitamin and mineral supplements cannot be used by the body and in general are excreted unused.

Whatever the scientific facts about the alternative therapies in cancer they do have one clear psychological advantage over conventional treatment. Patients feel they are being given back some control over their lives. They are offered some way of helping themselves instead of handing over their destiny to doctors and their high-tech treatments.

MOBILIZING YOUR NATURAL RESOURCES

The most well known and probably the largest place in Great Britain specializing in both the nutritional and psychological approach to treatment of people with cancer is the Bristol Cancer Help Centre. This opened in 1980 with the aims of stimulating a hopeful, positive attitude of mind in people with cancer and their relatives through a programme of healing, psychotherapy and dietary change supervised by doctors, nurses, counsellors, nutritionists and other therapists.

Central to the Bristol approach is the idea of 'energizing' the body to boost the immune system into renewing its protection of the body against cancer. They believe that in the healthy person defence cells in the blood routinely dispose of cells showing signs of turning cancerous. In cancer these defence cells decide to withdraw their protection and allow the tumour to take hold. At Bristol, the idea is to make the immune system take back responsibility for killing cancer cells. Doctors and therapists there believe it is possible to do this through a combination of dietary, emotional, psychological and spiritual changes. But just what do they mean by 'energizing' and is it really possible to switch on the immune system in this way?

Most of us think of energy in terms of whether we feel up to doing something. How often do we claim we just haven't got the energy to do the washing or the cleaning, to walk the dog or clean the car? Scientists take a rather more sophisticated approach to energy; they measure it in terms of what is available to do work. In physical terms we base the amount of energy we can expend in work on the amount of calories we take in through our food. We in the West take in far more calories than we really need for the physical and mental work which we do and these unnecessary calories weigh heavily on our waist-lines.

While it is quite easy to measure the number of calories or energy required to do a physical job it is virtually impossible to put a figure on mental energy. You can sit at a computer all day and not move a muscle in physical work but you can still come away from the terminal exhausted – 'drained of energy'.

This is the 'energy' which is important to the Bristol approach to treating cancer. Consider that indefinable 'energy' you get from going on holiday. Two weeks of good food and relaxation sends you back to work with a new vitality, a bloom on your skin and a spring in your step. It certainly isn't something you can define scientifically, but you do feel a surge of 'energy' which enables you to tackle your work much more easily than before you went on holiday. What they try to do at Bristol is to enable you to tap that energy to fight your cancer. As one of the Centre's therapists put it: 'It's like going on holiday, but much more profound.' How do they do it?

There are two options:

- Day-patients undergo a one-day introduction to the dietary, emotional and other healing techniques, with follow-up return days to reinforce and monitor how they are getting on.
- Residential patients stay for a one-week intensive residential course of therapy involving more detailed psychological therapy, followed by day return visits.

Central to both programmes is the Bristol Diet. Wherever possible this begins with a three-month 'clean-out' phase when people are encouraged to give up all meat, fish and dairy products. The idea is to cleanse the body of all the fats, refined products, chemicals and additives to be found in today's diet which those at Bristol believe to have lost their 'energy'. After the three-month period, some people remain vegetarian while others may add eggs, fish and poultry in moderation. Red and fatty meats such as beef, pork and lamb are strongly discouraged.

People on the Bristol programme learn about the diet and how to adapt their shopping, cooking and eating habits during the day or residential visits. They have one-hour-long counselling sessions, sometimes longer on the residential sessions. They learn breathing and relaxation techniques and they learn about imaging. This is a way of fighting the cancer by using gentle images of the immune system overcoming the tumour – sunshine melting ice, for example.

Many people, when asked to imagine what their cancer looks like, see it as some large, powerful and terrifying monster; their own defence cells they see as pathetic little creatures wandering aimlessly and helplessly around the monster cancer. The object of direct imaging is to swap these roles. Cancer cells are not the strong, clever creatures which many people think. Instead they are the weak ones, multiplying out of control, unable to repair the damage inflicted by anti-cancer drugs. Defence cells, on the other hand, are the clever ones, programmed to attack and fight invading marauders.

While those on day visits to Bristol learn the basics of diet, relaxation and imaging, those on the residential course are encouraged to explore much more about themselves – about the events and feelings they had in the months which preceded their diagnosis which may have contributed to the illness. They examine their own feelings towards their cancer and how these could be used more positively. Days three and four of the programme are crucial. Both begin like the other days with optional prayers and meditation, some aspect of the diet and gentle exercise. On day three this is followed by a lengthy session with the counsellor to find out what would 'energize' each individual mentally. We all know the sorts of things which give us greatest happiness or fulfilment – the things which 'make our hearts sing'. Again and again, the Bristol team has found that people who come to them for help have no song; sometimes they have lost it, often they never had one. They speak of lives full of disappointments and unfulfilled dreams. This isn't true of everyone who passes through the Bristol Centre. It may not be possible to identify anything which may have contributed to the lack of energy which triggered the cancer. But sometimes there is a major life crisis – bereavement, divorce, loss of a job – which preceded the discovery of the cancer. And with others a long-term feeling of helplessness may eventually have left the individual drained of reserves to fight the cancer when it turned up.

The purpose of this deeply emotional counselling session midway through the residential programme is to try and find out what may have helped trigger the cancer and, once identified, to consider how these feelings and attitudes might be changed. This process continues during the fourth day of the programme when once again counsellor and patient investigate the emotional, psychological and spiritual characteristics which are blocking the energy needed for recovery. Often there is an important outpouring of pent-up emotions such as rage and sorrow. Only by identifying these feelings can they be used in a positive rather than a negative way to fight the cancer.

This is, of necessity, only a very superficial account of the type of holistic approach taken by the Bristol Centre and, to a lesser degree, by other therapists. Such approaches are highly controversial. While accepting that there is some psychological input to any illness and that a positive outlook can significantly aid the response, few orthodox doctors can accept that the 'energizing' approach attributed to the dietary modification and psychological and spiritual healing can cure cancer. The Bristol group has modified its approach since the early days and many of the most controversial aspects of the programme such as coffee enemas and the drug, laetrile, have been replaced. Therapists have never seen their approach as a replacement for orthodox medicine but as complementary. Some of the people who have gone to the Bristol Centre have chosen to give up orthodox radiotherapy and chemotherapy; most have continued with their orthodox treatment.

As news of the Centre – and its more complementary approach – has spread, many orthodox specialists and GPs have suggested to their patients that they try the Centre. And anyone who goes is asked to sign a form confirming that they understand that they are not being encouraged to give up orthodox treatment.

Like any centre treating cancer patients, orthodox or complementary, there are those who have defied all the expectations of the doctors by living happy lives long after they should have been dead. And, inevitably, there are those who have died. Part of the Bristol approach is to prepare people for death – after all, no one is immortal. At Bristol, death is seen simply as the border between two worlds – packing up at the end of term for the school holidays, as one therapist put it; certainly not something to be feared.

A study of the methods used at Bristol is currently underway funded by the Imperial Cancer Research Fund and the Cancer Research Campaign. It falls into two parts. In the first it will try to find out whether the Bristol methods, with or without conventional treatment, can prolong life. The second and, to the Bristol team, more important part will try to analyse whether the Bristol methods improve the quality of life of the people who go through the programme. The results are unlikely to be as clear-cut as perhaps some scientists would like, but they should go some way to identifying the benefits and the drawbacks of the holistic approach to cancer treatment. Perhaps most important they demonstrate a long-awaited willingness by previously incompatible protagonists to examine the value of each other's methods towards a common goal.

Chapter Five

TYPES OF CANCER

HOW TO USE THIS CHAPTER

In this chapter we have provided a guide to the diagnosis and treatment of thirty of the most common types of cancer. We hope it will be a useful source of reference; it is geared mainly towards people who have symptoms which mean that cancer cannot be ruled out. They may have a lump or swelling, they may be losing weight and feeling unwell. Perhaps they are starting on a series of tests to find out just what is wrong with them.

We do stress that most of the symptoms described in this chapter are also common in many, many other illnesses which are nothing to do with cancer. Just because you have a headache it does not mean you have a brain tumour! Blood on the toilet paper is much more likely to mean that you have been straining too hard than that you have a bowel tumour! There are dozens of reasons why you could be losing weight and feeling feverish and off colour; it does not mean you have leukaemia! The same goes for lumps and swellings – the vast majority are benign and not cancers, frequently just watery cysts.

But you should not ignore them. The only way to find out why you are getting symptoms is to examine you and carry out a series of tests, some at the GP's surgery, some at hospital. Your symptoms are only one piece of the jig-saw. Put in the results of the other investigations and you could end up with a totally different picture from the one you expected from your symptoms.

Nearly all the diagnostic tests described in this chapter are used to identify diseases other than cancer. Blood tests, X-rays, scans, and all the 'scope' tests which involve putting flexible tubes up or down the hollow passage-ways of the body are used routinely in all areas of medicine. Just because your neighbour had a bone scan and she had cancer it does not mean that your bone scan will find the same thing. Most of the tests will be done to exclude diseases rather than specifically to find them. Thus, if you have a pain in your chest, there will be tests to exclude heart and digestive problems as well as to see whether there is a shadow on your lung X-ray.

It is inevitable that some people who have these tests will be found to have cancer and we hope that this chapter will be useful to them too. For each cancer, we have described the options which are available for treatment. This does not mean that you will get exactly what is described here. We have deliberately not included drug names where treatment involves chemotherapy as these vary from hospital to hospital. The same goes for doses of radiotherapy, which are tailored to individual people. Cancer specialists are constantly experimenting with new drugs and new combinations of treatment and so what is described in this book can only be a guide. Just because you are not getting what is included here does not mean that you are not getting good treatment, though you should remember that if you are unhappy you can ask to be referred for a second opinion.

Most people who are diagnosed with cancer do ask what is likely to happen to them. It is often difficult for doctors to predict how they will respond to treatment and whether they can be cured. But since so many people do ask, we have included a section on follow-up and long-term outcome for each cancer. We have tried to give some idea of what to expect, based on current statistics. Cure rates are much better for some cancers than they were even ten to fifteen years ago and progress is being made all the time. The figures which we have given are a guide and a lot will depend on how early the cancer is diagnosed, how aggressively you decide it should be treated, your age and the general state of your health.

The cancers discussed in this chapter are grouped together according to whether they occur in adults or children, and are listed roughly in order of decreasing frequency.

LUNG CANCER

DESCRIPTION

4 main types:
1. Squamous cell
2. Small (oat) cell
3. Large cell
4. Adenocarcinoma

Most start in main air tubes to lungs and spread. Small cell tumours are fastest growing.

SYMPTOMS

1. Chronic cough with or without blood
2. Chronic chest infection
3. Hoarseness
4. Chest pain

DIAGNOSIS

What the GP may do
1. General physical examination

What the specialist may do
1. X-rays
2. Bronchoscopy or surgery for biopsy
3. Breathing tests
4. Hormone tests (can confirm small cell tumour)
5. Scans for secondaries

TREATMENT

Small cell tumours: chemotherapy and possibly radiotherapy
Other tumours: surgery for small accessible tumours or radiotherapy and/or chemotherapy

FOLLOW-UP
AND OUTLOOK

Tend to spread to bone, brain and liver. Only 6 per cent cure rate; most die within one year of diagnosis. Biggest cancer killer in the UK. 40 000 deaths per year – 90 per cent caused by smoking cigarettes and therefore preventable.

BOWEL CANCER

DESCRIPTION   Two areas:
1. Large intestine (colon) – more common in women
2. Rectum – more common in men

Both more common in countries where diet is low in fibre and high in animal fat and refined carbohydrate.

SYMPTOMS   1. Blood in faeces
2. Chronic change in bowel habit to diarrhoea or constipation
3. Abdominal pain and weight loss

DIAGNOSIS   *What the GP may do*
1. Ask for faeces sample for laboratory tests
2. Examine rectum

What the specialist may do
1. Full physical and rectal examination
2. Barium enema X-ray
3. Colonoscopy or sigmoidoscopy for biopsy

TREATMENT   1. Surgery to remove tumour or section of bowel. This may mean a colostomy so that faeces are passed through an opening made in the surface of the abdomen
2. Sometimes follow-up drugs or radiotherapy are given

FOLLOW-UP   Depends how early tumour is diagnosed. One
AND OUTLOOK   third cured by surgery.
Tends to spread to liver.
High-fibre diet may reduce the risk of getting bowel cancer but cannot affect established cancer.

BREAST CANCER

DESCRIPTION
Affects about one woman in 17, mainly over the age of 50.
Tumours start in milk ducts and spread.
More common on outer edge of breast than along cleavage line.

SYMPTOMS
Lump (NB most lumps are not cancer)
Pain in breast
Change in breast shape
Blood or discharge from nipple

DIAGNOSIS
What the GP may do
1. Examine breasts and glands under arms and in neck

What the specialist may do
1. Breast examination
2. Breast X-ray (mammography)
3. Biopsy:
   (i) with a needle in out-patients
   (ii) under general anaesthetic as in-patient

TREATMENT
1. Lumpectomy or mastectomy depending on size, extent and position of tumour
2. Radiotherapy: commonly after lumpectomy to prevent recurrence in the breast
3. Chemotherapy: if tumour has spread to lymph nodes
4. Hormones: (e.g. tamoxifen) for recurrence or to prevent spread
5. Removal of ovaries – for recurrence

FOLLOW-UP AND OUTLOOK
Tends to spread to bones and spine. Number of sufferers living five to ten years is increasing.

STOMACH CANCER

DESCRIPTION Tends to occur in lower part of stomach where it joins the intestine.
More common in men than in women, especially in younger age-groups.

SYMPTOMS 1. Indigestion
2. Pain in upper abdomen
3. Sometimes vomiting of blood
4. Loss of weight and appetite

DIAGNOSIS *What the GP may do*
1. Full physical examination

What the specialist may do
1. Barium meal X-ray
2. Gastroscopy to get biopsy sample

TREATMENT 1. Surgery to remove small, localized tumours and part of stomach
2. Palliative surgery to relieve symptoms if tumour has spread
3. Radiotherapy for pain if tumour has spread
4. Sometimes chemotherapy

FOLLOW-UP AND OUTLOOK Tends to spread to liver.
Outlook poor unless caught early.

PROSTATE CANCER

DESCRIPTION
All men have some prostate enlargement with age. Sometimes this is due to a tumour which can block the passage of urine from the bladder.

SYMPTOMS
1. Trouble passing urine
2. Pain on passing urine
3. Sometimes the passing of blood
4. Bone pain (especially backache) if tumour has already spread

DIAGNOSIS
What the GP may do
1. Examine prostate by putting finger into rectum
2. Take blood samples (for laboratory tests)

What the specialist may do
1. Examination and biopsy
2. X-rays and scans (with radioactive substance) for secondaries
3. Take blood samples

TREATMENT
Depends on age as tumours grow slowly and normal life-expectancy may not be great:
1. Radiotherapy
2. Surgery, but this is a major operation with significant risk of mortality and impotence
3. Female hormones to relieve pain and urine obstruction if tumour has spread
4. Or remove testicles for the same reason
5. Or drugs to block male hormones

FOLLOW-UP
AND OUTLOOK
Tends to spread to bone.
Unless caught early the chances of cure are small, but because it is a cancer of older men and tumours grow slowly death may occur from other causes.

PANCREATIC CANCER

DESCRIPTION Tumours generally start in the ducts carrying pancreatic juices for food digestion; very rarely they occur in the islet cells which make insulin to control blood sugar levels.

SYMPTOMS
1. Abdominal pain and discomfort, backache
2. Loss of appetite and weight loss

DIAGNOSIS *What the GP may do*
1. Physical examination

What the specialist may do
1. Barium meal X-ray
2. Ultrasound, computerized tomography (CT) scan of abdomen
3. Blood tests
4. Exploratory operation to get biopsy material for examination under the microscope

TREATMENT
1. Palliative surgery to unblock the bile duct
2. If cancer restricted to the pancreas the organ may be removed (rarely possible)
3. Radiotherapy or chemotherapy to relieve symptoms

FOLLOW-UP AND OUTLOOK The outlook is not good but survival varies enormously from a few months to years, depending on the extent of the disease when it is diagnosed.

BLADDER CANCER

DESCRIPTION   Occurs mainly in older people and is more common in men than women and in people who smoke.

SYMPTOMS
1. Blood in the urine
2. Pain in the lower abdomen
3. Need to pass urine frequently
4. Pain in passing urine

DIAGNOSIS   *What the GP may do*
1. Physical examination
2. Asks for urine sample for laboratory tests

What the specialist may do
1. X-rays, generally with dye (intravenous pyelogram (IVP))
2. CT or ultrasound scan
3. Cystoscopy to see inside of the bladder and to get biopsy sample

TREATMENT
1. Surgery: this will depend on type, size and spread of tumour
2. Radiotherapy or chemotherapy in some cases

FOLLOW-UP AND OUTLOOK   Tends to spread to liver, lungs and bones.
Survival depends on type and extent of tumour.
Recurrences common.

OESOPHAGEAL CANCER

DESCRIPTION The oesophagus is the tube which carries food from the mouth to the stomach. Tumours start in the wall of the tube and grow into the hollow passage, eventually causing an obstruction.

SYMPTOMS
1. Increasing difficulty with swallowing
2. Pain and discomfort in chest
3. Loss of appetite and weight

DIAGNOSIS *What the GP may do*
1. Check symptoms to ensure that pain and discomfort are not due to circulatory disease
2. Antacids may be prescribed to see if these relieve symptoms

What the specialist may do
1. Barium meal X-rays
2. Endoscopy to examine inside of oesophagus and obtain biopsy for examination under the microscope
3. Other X-rays and scans to see if cancer has spread

TREATMENT
1. Surgery to remove the tumour if it is in the lower part of the oesophagus. This can be cut out and the bottom end rejoined to the stomach
2. If tumour has spread, palliative surgery to reduce blockage and make patient more comfortable
3. Radiotherapy to reduce size of tumour if it is inaccessible surgically

FOLLOW-UP AND OUTLOOK Unfortunately, like most tumours of the gastro-intestinal tract, oesophageal cancer is rarely detected until it has spread from its initial site – generally to lymph nodes and then to the liver. So prognosis is poor.

OVARIAN CANCER

DESCRIPTION Occurs in either or both ovaries, mainly in women aged 40–60, especially if childless. Most common tumour of female reproductive tract.

SYMPTOMS Very vague; possibly:
1. Swelling in abdomen
2. Nausea, indigestion or constipation

DIAGNOSIS *What the GP may do*
1. External and internal examination

What the specialist may do
1. Physical examination
2. Ultrasound, body scan
3. Biopsy
4. Exploratory operation

TREATMENT
1. Surgery to remove both ovaries and womb. Occasionally it may be possible to save one ovary and the womb if the woman especially wants children, but this is generally inadvisable
2. Chemotherapy for recurrences. Sometimes radiotherapy
3. Chemotherapy for advanced disease

FOLLOW-UP AND OUTLOOK
Tends to spread to abdominal organs.
Long-term outlook depends on how early the tumour is diagnosed (most are diagnosed late because of lack of symptoms).
Cure rate poor but better drugs (based on platinum) are improving survival rates.

ADULT LEUKAEMIA

DESCRIPTION

Two categories:
1. Acute
2. Chronic

All leukaemias affect the cells produced in the bone marrow which make up the red and white cells of the blood; the name of each variety refers to the particular group of cells which is affected. Acute myeloblastic leukaemia is the most common form.

SYMPTOMS

Rather vague and related to the type of blood cell which is affected. Thus:

1. Low levels of white cells – repeated infections
2. Lack of platelet cells – excessive bruising or bleeding from gums
3. Low levels of red cells: tiredness and generally feeling unwell
4. Enlarged lymph nodes

DIAGNOSIS

What the GP may do
1. Physical examination, especially of lymph glands, liver and spleen
2. Take blood samples for laboratory tests

What the specialist may do
1. More blood and bone marrow tests
2. Samples of lymph node cells taken

TREATMENT

Precise treatment plans vary from centre to centre.
Acute myeloblastic leukaemia: chemotherapy. Bone marrow transplant in young people if suitable donor can be found.

Acute lymphocytic leukaemia: chemotherapy, with radiotherapy to head. Bone marrow transplant as second-line treatment if suitable donor can be found. More chemotherapy.

Chronic myeloblastic leukaemia: chemotherapy. A small proportion of young patients can be cured with bone marrow transplant if suitable donor available.

Chronic lymphoblastic leukaemia: chemotherapy, which is less aggressive than for other types. This is to reduce symptoms rather than to cure. Some patients need no treatment for many years.

FOLLOW-UP
AND OUTLOOK

Very careful monitoring of blood and bone marrow are needed so that new courses of chemotherapy can start at the first sign of recurrence.

Prospects for those with acute leukaemias have improved dramatically in recent years.

People with chronic leukaemias are not cured but may live a long time.

HODGKIN'S DISEASE AND NON-HODGKIN'S LYMPHOMAS

DESCRIPTION Distinguished by appearance under micro-scope. All are tumours of lymphatic system – a series of fine tubes which link nodes and get rid of excess fluid in tissues and produce some defence cells. Main nodes are in neck, under arms, in the middle of the chest and along the main blood vessels in abdomen.

SYMPTOMS 1. Persistent painless swelling in one or more lymph nodes, sometimes accompanied by:
  1. general tiredness
  2. weight loss
  3. night sweats and fevers
  4. itching

DIAGNOSIS *What the GP may do*
  1. Physical examination especially of lymph nodes
  2. Take blood samples for laboratory tests

What the specialist may do
  1. Biopsy from lymph nodes under general anaesthetic for examination under micro-scope
  2. X-rays
  3. Ultrasound and CT scans of abdomen (often with dye)
  4. Occasionally an exploratory abdominal operation may be done in the case of Hodgkin's disease

TREATMENT

Radiotherapy and/or chemotherapy are used for both forms of the disease. But the exact treatment depends on the type of lymphoma and the extent of spread.

Chemotherapy can be effective for even advanced Hodgkin's disease.

FOLLOW-UP AND OUTLOOK

Treatment of Hodgkin's disease is one of the big success stories in cancer and around two-thirds of people are cured with others having long remissions and prolonged survival. Cure rates for non-Hodgkin's disease are lower but there is a good chance of a long remission.

BRAIN TUMOURS

DESCRIPTION The brain is a common site for secondary tumours which have spread from other organs. Most primary brain tumours are gliomas – so called because they develop in the supporting tissue of the nervous system, rather than from the nerve cells themselves. Benign tumours, or meningiomas, may occur at the surface of the brain. Adult brain tumours are most common in the 30–60 age-group.

SYMPTOMS These vary and depend on where the tumour is sited and the function of the brain tissue on which it is pressing.
1. Severe persistent headaches which increase in severity (NB brain tumours are a very rare cause of headaches)
2. Seizures and epileptic fits
3. Nausea and vomiting
4. Confusion

DIAGNOSIS *What the GP may do*
1. Careful assessment of the importance of what may seem to be unrelated physical, nervous and psychological symptoms

What the specialist may do
1. X-rays and scans with dyes to get best pictures
2. Recordings of electrical activity in the brain (EEGs)

TREATMENT 1. Surgery if the tumour is accessible
2. Radiotherapy if surgery is likely to do too much damage to surrounding tissues
3. Radiotherapy following surgery to get rid of remaining cancer cells

4. Chemotherapy to shrink tumours before surgery or to prevent spread afterwards

FOLLOW-UP AND OUTLOOK

Cure depends on the type of brain tumour, but people can survive many years after tumours are removed. If they spread this tends to be to other nervous tissues in the body. Prognosis for those with benign tumours is good provided they can be removed and prevented from pressing on surrounding tissue.

CANCER OF THE KIDNEY

DESCRIPTION
This occurs more often in men than women and, though rare, is more likely to occur over the age of 50. It is much more common in smokers.

SYMPTOMS
1. Blood in the urine
2. Pain in the back or on passing urine
3. Tiredness and feeling generally unwell
4. Unexplained fever

DIAGNOSIS
What the GP may do
1. Physical examination especially checking for signs of swelling over the kidney
2. Send urine sample for laboratory tests

What the specialist may do
1. X-rays with dye for best pictures – intravenous pyelogram (IVP)
2. Ultrasound or CT scans

TREATMENT
1. Surgical removal of tumour if small or of whole kidney if larger
2. Radiotherapy for secondaries in bone

FOLLOW-UP AND OUTLOOK
Kidney tumours tend to spread to bone and brain tissue. If the cancer is confined to the kidney cure is possible by surgical removal. Long-term outlook is less good if the tumour has already spread.

CERVICAL CANCER

DESCRIPTION   Results from a series of changes in the cells of the neck of the womb. Early changes are pre-malignant and can be picked up with smear tests and monitored. Sometimes pre-malignant changes revert to normal or they may develop so that treatment is needed to prevent cancer itself.

SYMPTOMS   Ideally, cervical cancer – or the pre-malignant changes which precede it – should be picked up before symptoms occur. But in the later stages symptoms are:
1. Vaginal discharge
2. Pain
3. Bleeding

DIAGNOSIS   *What the GP may do*
1. Vaginal examination
2. Take cervical smear for laboratory tests

What the specialist may do
1. Physical examination
2. Further cervical samples
3. Dilatation and curettage (D and C) to check how far the tumour has spread into the cervix and womb
4. X-rays and ultrasound for further signs of spread

TREATMENT   Depends on extent of disease:
1. Laser, heat or cold treatment for earliest pre-malignant changes
2. Surgical removal of wedge of cancerous tissue if more advanced
3. Hysterectomy for more advanced disease to remove cervix, womb and possibly ovaries

and Fallopian tubes depending on spread of cancer
4. Radiotherapy as an alternative to hysterectomy
5. Chemotherapy

FOLLOW-UP AND OUTLOOK

Regardless of treatment, samples of cells will need to be taken from the cervix to check for recurrence.

If treated early, before changes become malignant, most women are cured by laser therapy. The prospects are far less good for women diagnosed late.

MULTIPLE MYELOMA

DESCRIPTION Another disease of the bone marrow cells, affecting the plasma cells which make antibodies to combat infection. It is most common in middle or old age.

SYMPTOMS 1. Recurrent infection which does not respond to antibiotics
2. Bone pain
3. Loss of energy

DIAGNOSIS *What the GP may do*
1. Physical examination to exclude other conditions
2. Take blood samples for laboratory tests

What the specialist may do
1. More blood and bone marrow tests
2. X-rays to see if cancer is in the bones

TREATMENT 1. Chemotherapy to combat the cancer
2. Supportive treatment to relieve or prevent symptoms, e.g. reduction of calcium levels resulting from bone damage
3. Radiotherapy to relieve bone pain

FOLLOW-UP AND OUTLOOK Initially, treatment will keep the cancer at bay and supportive measures will prevent painful symptoms. Long-term outlook is less good but since the disease tends to occur in older people the loss of life-expectancy is not as great as if the disease was common in young people. More intensive treatments are being developed for younger people and these may be associated with a better outlook.

LIVER CANCER

DESCRIPTION The liver is a common site for secondary tumours of cancers from other organs. But cancer starting in the liver is rare in Europe and North America. Liver cancer occurs more often in men, though women's livers are more susceptible to alcohol damage.

SYMPTOMS
1. Pain and discomfort in the abdomen
2. Loss of weight and appetite
3. Jaundice
4. Bloated abdomen

DIAGNOSIS *What the GP may do*
1. Physical examination: the liver may feel hard or bloated to the touch

What the specialist may do
1. Barium meal X-rays
2. Ultrasound and CT scans
3. Blood tests for liver function

TREATMENT
1. Surgery if tumours are confined to one part of the liver and can be removed, but this is rare.
2. Radiotherapy and/or chemotherapy to help relieve symptoms

FOLLOW-UP AND OUTLOOK Outlook is poor, though survival can vary.

CANCER OF THE UTERUS

DESCRIPTION Most cancers start in the inner lining of the womb, or uterus. Much more common than cancer are benign lumps in the womb, called fibroids. Cancer is more likely to occur in older women, after the menopause. Uterine cancer is the least common of the cancers of the female reproductive tract.

SYMPTOMS 1. Bleeding from the vagina (since most women are post-menopausal when they develop uterine cancer this symptom is not generally confused with normal menstruation)

DIAGNOSIS *What the GP may do*
1. Vaginal and cervical examination
2. Cervical smear for laboratory tests to see if cancerous cells have come down from the womb and lodged on the cervix

What the specialist may do
1. Dilatation and curettage (D and C) to get cells from the inside of the womb
2. Blood tests
3. X-rays and scans

TREATMENT 1. Surgery to remove the womb and the ovaries and Fallopian tubes in case the cancer has spread upwards.
2. Radiotherapy if the tumour has grown deeper into the wall of the womb
3. Hormone treatment for advanced or recurrent disease since many uterine tumours are sensitive to the female hormone, progesterone

FOLLOW-UP
AND OUTLOOK
Most women found to have early uterine cancer are cured. Uterine cancer tends to spread to the lungs, bones, liver and brain. Of those where the tumour has spread widely into the uterine muscle and require radiotherapy, about half will be cured. When the tumour has spread further the results are less good, though hormone treatment can prolong survival.

SKIN CANCER

DESCRIPTION
Three main types; in order of increasing severity:
1. Basal cell, or rodent ulcer
2. Squamous cell
3. Malignant melanoma

All are most common in fair-skinned people who are exposed to prolonged harsh sunlight. So skin cancer is especially common in Australia, and malignant melanoma, though still rare, is increasing in the UK.

SYMPTOMS
Seen rather than felt.
1. Basal cell starts as a firm, waxy lump whose centre ulcerates.
2. Squamous cell appears hard and scaly and may ulcerate, often with a scab.
3. Malignant melanoma may start in a mole or birthmark but can arise in normal unmarked skin. Look for uneven edge, rough surface, change in colour or increase in size.
4. Bleeding is a late symptom.

DIAGNOSIS
What the GP may do
1. Skin examination to rule out other conditions

What the specialist may do
1. Take skin sample for examination under microscope
2. Investigate to see if the tumour has spread

TREATMENT
1. Surgery: small incision under local anaesthetic for basal or squamous cell
2. Electro- or cryosurgery to burn or freeze off small tumours

3. Radiotherapy for larger tumours or where surgery would be disfiguring
4. Malignant melanoma: more radical surgery to remove tumour and surrounding skin. Removal of lymph nodes if tumour has spread to them
5. Chemotherapy to relieve symptoms (rarely prolongs life)

FOLLOW-UP AND OUTLOOK

Rodent ulcers and squamous cell tumours are almost always cured by surgery. The prospects for someone with malignant melanoma depend on how quickly it is treated and whether it has spread. Secondary tumours tend to occur in the chest, liver, bone and brain. Even so, long remissions are possible.

VAGINAL AND VULVAL CANCERS

DESCRIPTION   These are rare genital cancers. Tumours of the vagina and the vulva, the opening to the vagina, tend to occur in older women.

SYMPTOMS   Vulval cancer:
1. Persistent irritation at vaginal opening and sometimes pain

Vaginal cancer:
1. Vaginal discharge
2. Abnormal bleeding
3. Pain

DIAGNOSIS   *What the GP may do*
1. Genital examination for lump
2. Vaginal or vulval cell samples sent for laboratory tests
3. Blood samples sent for laboratory tests

What the specialist may do
1. Check results of laboratory tests and GP's initial examination
2. X-rays and scans for signs of secondaries

TREATMENT   1. Vulval tumours are removed surgically
2. Vaginal tumours respond well to radiotherapy

FOLLOW-UP AND OUTLOOK   Cure rates for vaginal cancer are less good than for vulval cancer but a lot depends on how early the tumour is caught and treated.

CHORIOCARCINOMA

DESCRIPTION Choriocarcinoma occurs in young women as it is a cancer of the placenta. It can occur after a pregnancy, miscarriage or abortion

SYMPTOMS 1. Continuous bleeding after pregnancy
2. Symptoms from secondary tumours in the chest (e.g. breathing problems) because the tumour grows so fast

DIAGNOSIS *What the GP may do*
1. Internal vaginal examination
2. Blood samples sent for laboratory tests

What the specialist may do
1. Check results of laboratory tests and GP's initial examination
2. X-rays and scans for signs of secondary tumours

TREATMENT 1. Chemotherapy

FOLLOW-UP The outlook for women with choriocarcinoma
AND OUTLOOK has been dramatically improved in the last 30 years and there is a good chance of cure.

TESTICULAR CANCER

DESCRIPTION   Two common types, roughly equal in frequency:
1. Seminoma – more common in 30–40 age-group
2. Teratoma – more common in 15–30 age-group

Account for 2 per cent of male cancers but most common cancer in young men. Occur more often in men who had undescended testicles as children.

SYMPTOMS   1. Swelling in testicle which may or may not be painful
2. Back pain

DIAGNOSIS   *What the GP may do*
1. Examine testicles and do more general physical examination

What the specialist may do
1. Exploratory operation to remove testicle for examination under microscope
2. Blood tests to confirm whether seminoma or teratoma (teratoma produces alpha fetoprotein (AFP) and higher levels of human chorionic gonadotrophin (HCG) than seminoma)
3. X-rays and scans to check for spread

TREATMENT   1. Surgery to remove affected testicle and to make diagnosis
2. Seminoma: if tumour confined to testis, either careful follow-up or radiotherapy to abdominal lymph nodes. Chemotherapy if tumour more advanced.

3. Teratoma: if tumour confined to testis either careful follow-up or chemotherapy. All other stages get chemotherapy, sometimes backed up by surgery to bulky lymph nodes

FOLLOW-UP AND OUTLOOK

Testicular cancer, especially teratoma which had the poorer results, has been one of the success stories of recent years. In the last 20 years survival rates have shot up from less than 50 per cent to over 90 per cent.

HEAD AND NECK CANCER

DESCRIPTION
A range of tumours can occur in the head and neck, including the mouth, salivary glands, nose, air passage, voice box and throat. Tumours tend to occur more often in older people, over 60.

SYMPTOMS
These depend very much on the site of the tumour:
1. Breathing difficulties, cough
2. Lump or swelling
3. Hoarseness
4. Swallowing difficulties

DIAGNOSIS
What the GP may do
1. Physical examination of the inside of nose and mouth

What the specialist may do
1. X-rays, CT and ultrasound scans of relevant areas. Barium swallow may be used to improve pictures

TREATMENT
1. Surgery geared to removal of maximum amount of tumour with minimum disfigurement
2. Radiotherapy where more appropriate
3. Sometimes chemotherapy to shrink tumours before surgery

FOLLOW-UP AND OUTLOOK
Since head and neck tumours tend to occur in older people survival may not be substantially less than expected.
Tumours tend to spread to the lymph nodes in the neck and take some time to form secondaries elsewhere in the body.

CHILDHOOD CANCERS

LEUKAEMIA

DESCRIPTION There are several different types, each affecting the bone marrow which produces red and white blood cells and platelets. By far the most common form in childhood is acute lymphoblastic leukaemia (ALL) which accounts for about one in three of all cancers in children

SYMPTOMS Rather vague and related to which bone marrow cells are affected:
1. Tiredness, pallor and feeling unwell
2. Shortness of breath
3. Frequent infections
4. Platelets affected – bruising and bleeding

DIAGNOSIS *What the GP may do*
1. Blood tests
2. Physical examination

What the specialist may do
1. Bone marrow tests
2. Further blood tests

TREATMENT 1. Intensive chemotherapy
2. Supportive treatment, including blood transfusions, antibiotics, etc. as required
Acute lymphoblastic leukaemia: radiotherapy to prevent spread of cancer into brain and spinal cord. Low-dose maintenance chemotherapy to keep child in remission.
Treatment is begun again if relapse occurs. Bone marrow transplant may be attempted during second remission after first relapse if suitable donor can be found, or in first remission for acute myeloblastic leukaemia.

FOLLOW-UP
AND OUTLOOK

Treatment of childhood leukaemia has been one of the real success stories of cancer with a 50 per cent cure rate, thanks to modern drugs and support therapy.

BONE SARCOMAS

DESCRIPTION There are three main types:
1. Osteosarcoma – mainly affects limb bones of boys and young men aged 10–25
2. Ewing's sarcoma – occurs in any bone, mainly in children aged 5–16
3. Chondrosarcoma – is the least serious bone tumour and often develops from a benign lump

Tumours of muscle and connective tissue are rarer and tend to be lumped together as soft tissue sarcomas.

SYMPTOMS 1. Bone pain
2. Bone swelling
3. Sometimes movement problems and fractures
4. Fever

DIAGNOSIS *What the GP may do*
1. Physical examination to exclude other causes of pain or swelling such as sport or other injuries

What the specialist may do
1. X-rays and bone scans
2. Biopsy of bone lump for examination under microscope
3. Blood tests and occasionally bone marrow samples for laboratory tests

TREATMENT *Osteosarcoma*: chemotherapy followed by surgery followed by more chemotherapy. Sometimes amputation is necessary, or it may be enough to remove a section of bone and replace it with a metal prosthesis.

Ewing's sarcoma: chemotherapy and radio-therapy. Amputation or surgical replacement of bone are sometimes needed.
Chondrosarcoma: surgery.

FOLLOW-UP
AND OUTLOOK

The highest cure rate is achieved with chon-drosarcoma where surgical removal of the tumour may be all that is needed. Cure rates for osteosarcoma and Ewing's sarcoma are up to 40 per cent.

NEUROBLASTOMA

DESCRIPTION Neuroblastoma forms from nerves of the sympathetic nervous system, which is responsible for activities over which we have no control, such as heart beat and bowel movement. They can occur anywhere in the body but are most common in the abdomen in the adrenal gland, above the kidney.

SYMPTOMS
1. Lump or swelling
2. Neuroblastoma secretes chemicals which may raise blood pressure

DIAGNOSIS *What the GP may do*
1. Physical examination for lumps
2. Take blood samples for laboratory tests

What the specialist may do
1. X-rays, with dyes to get best pictures
2. Scans
3. Urine tests for chemicals released by neuroblastoma
4. Bone marrow biopsy to check for spread

TREATMENT
1. Surgical removal of the tumour and chemotherapy
2. Radiotherapy for tumours which are inaccessible for surgery
The order in which these are used varies with the clinical problem. Most start with chemotherapy. A few can be cured by surgery alone.

FOLLOW-UP AND OUTLOOK Prospects are far better than even a decade ago. Carefully planned treatment has improved survival but this depends on how quickly the tumours are diagnosed.

WILMS' TUMOUR

DESCRIPTION

This starts in the kidney and is also called nephroblastoma

SYMPTOMS

1. Lump or swelling in the abdomen
2. Blood in urine
3. Fever
4. Abdominal discomfort

DIAGNOSIS

What the GP may do
1. General physical examination
2. Take blood samples for laboratory tests

What the specialist may do
1. X-rays, probably with injected dyes to get best pictures
2. Scans

TREATMENT

1. Surgical removal of the affected kidney
2. Follow-up chemotherapy, sometimes with radiotherapy

FOLLOW-UP AND OUTLOOK

Prospects are excellent.

Chapter Six

COPING WITH THE SIDE-EFFECTS OF YOUR TREATMENT

Just because you are being treated for cancer does not mean that you will suffer from any or all of the problems discussed in this chapter. No treatment for any medical condition is without its side-effects but, realistically, people who are treated for cancer have more than their fair share of side-effects.

However, there are ways of minimizing many of these problems if you know how. We have divided this chapter into three: chemotherapy, radiotherapy and surgery. Each section deals with the problems most likely to arise with these forms of treatment. There is some overlap. For example, many people with cancer have trouble eating – regardless of the type of treatment they are having. And at times you are likely to feel tired whether you have had surgery or are having a course of radiotherapy or chemotherapy. So we have discussed the best way of dealing with these problems under the type of treatment where they are most likely to occur.

Many of the problems which can arise with surgery are not typical only of operations for cancer. So rather than write a textbook of surgery we have discussed only the difficulties you may experience after some of the operations carried out most commonly in cancer: colostomies, mastectomies, hysterectomies and laryngectomies.

We hope that the information will be useful, but don't forget that the organizations which have been formed to provide support for people after these operations all produce detailed leaflets which may well contain the answers to questions which you may still have. Some hospitals have also put together information leaflets describing your treatment, its side-effects and how to cope with them, so it's worth asking about what is available.

Of course, the doctors and nurses who are giving you your treatment can also advise on coping with side-effects. Remember, whatever you are suffering from they will have seen it before. And no question you ask about your treatment should be too trivial for them to answer.

CHEMOTHERAPY

WHAT TO DO IF YOU CAN'T EAT

Many people with cancer find they have trouble eating – not just those on anti-cancer drugs. It is important to keep up your food intake because you can quickly lose large amounts of weight. But cancer and weight loss do not have to go together. There are lots of things you can do to boost your calorie intake without forcing yourself to eat large meals.

Some people believe that by eating they are feeding their tumour and helping it to grow. It is true that tumours do use extra energy, but they will take that from your body whether or not you are eating well. So at least if you are eating you can keep up your body's reserves of calories – and your strength to fight the cancer.

Anyone who has ever had trouble eating, for whatever reason, knows how off-putting it can be when some well-meaning friend or relative puts a large plate of meat and two veg in front of you along with the words 'That'll build you up.' Your heart sinks as you move the food about and try and make a few spaces between the mounds of veggies to suggest that you have eaten something.

When you are having trouble eating you want to get the maximum number of calories into you in the minimum amount of food. Any regular dieter can tell you about the vast amount of calories packed into nuts, for example, or chocolate bars. You also want something which does not require a great deal of chewing and will slip down easily, which is why soups, jellies and ice-cream are useful. This doesn't mean that your whole diet should be one continuous binge of sweet, fatty foods. It is as important for someone with cancer to eat a balanced diet as anyone else and that means a mix of protein, fat, carbohydrate and fibre.

It is just that instead of taking your protein through large lumps of red meat you may find thin slices of chicken breast more appetizing. Lightly grilled fish is likely to be far more tempting than cod in thick batter. Or you may prefer to leave fish and meat altogether and stick to eggs, soft cheese and milk instead.

In spite of the need to boost your calorie intake the key to success is small portions. You can always go back for more, but a packed plate will put you off before you even start.

Here are some tips to consider when preparing your meals or asking someone else to do them for you.

Breakfast

- Try drinking half a glass of concentrated orange juice while you are preparing breakfast; that way it won't stare at you from a queue of things to get through when you sit down to breakfast.
- Choose a cereal which comes in small pieces and does not take a lot of chewing. Avoid cereals with sharp corners which might catch on sore mouth ulcers.
- Use cream or the 'top of the milk' on your cereal and just take a couple of teaspoons of cereal if that's all you feel like.
- If you have coffee with your breakfast, make it with hot milk instead of with water. Not only will it give you extra calories and protein, it will probably go down more easily than stronger coffee which may irritate your stomach. In fact, make coffee as weak as you like.
- Avoid fatty 'fry-up' breakfasts unless you really fancy some eggs and bacon. Go instead for a boiled egg with a thin slice of toast, cut into 'soldiers'. Scrambled egg also goes down easily or an omelette if you fancy a change.
- If toast takes too much chewing just have bread and butter, cut into bite-sized 'postage stamps'.

Mid-morning snack

- Try a cup of milky coffee or, if you are very fond of milk, try half a glass on its own.

- Get in a supply of your favourite biscuits – you can always 'dunk' them if they are hard to chew!
- Keep a bag of small, soft-centred sweets to hand throughout the day and have one whenever you fancy it. Or, if you prefer savoury things, keep a few bowls of nuts or cheeselets around to dip into.
- Don't be afraid of 'spoiling your appetite'; eat a little of what you want, when you want.

Lunchtime

You may prefer to eat your main meal of the day at lunchtime because it is easier to digest than in the evening. Or you may like to vary it. For your main meal try to take in a small portion of each of the important components for a healthy diet.

- Meat: grill or bake meat rather than frying – you will find it easier to digest. Tasty sauces can liven up the meat and add a few extra calories. If you don't feel like making the sauce yourself, try one of the ready-made variety. Casseroles are a good idea because you can add beans or noodles for extra protein, and cream or a little wine for extra calories.
- Potatoes: mashed potato is always easiest to eat, provided it isn't hard or lumpy! Add milk or cream and butter to make it softer and richer but avoid getting it mushy and unappetizing. Croquette potatoes make a nice change and you can buy them ready-made to put in the oven or shallow fry. Baked potatoes are very nutritious, especially with the skins on. Choose small potatoes which are likely to have softest skins and put on a good dollop of butter or cheese before serving to make them moist.
- Other vegetables: never overcook, but this probably isn't the time to experiment with *la nouvelle cuisine*! Semi-raw vegetables are difficult to chew for someone with a sore mouth. Peas, sweetcorn and beans are a good idea because of their small size. But if you choose spinach or cabbage chop it up small. Pureed carrots, swedes or parsnips slip down more easily than the solid variety.
- Rice and pasta: these are high both in calorie-giving carbohydrates and in fibre and they make a tasty and easy-to-cook alternative to potatoes. Many pasta dishes include high-calorie

sauces involving cream or butter; try dishes such as pasta with butter and herbs and pasta with bacon, mushrooms and cream rather than the very rich tomato and meat sources which may be rather off-putting to the small appetite.

- Puddings: there is a wide range of packaged foods which can be made up with milk – rice puddings, semolinas, blancmanges, Instant Whips, Angel Delights and so on. They are a lot easier to eat than stodgy puddings and can easily have energy supplements added to them. Old favourites such as jellies and ice-creams are good stand-bys (some people find ice-cream too cold, others find it soothing). Pureed fruit with cream also goes down well.

Mid-afternoon snacks

This is a good time to tempt even the most difficult appetite with cakes and biscuits with the afternoon tea. But don't expect the large rich, cream-packed chocolate éclairs and meringues to disappear. Go for small, simple sponge cakes, perhaps with a little fancy icing – they are less challenging to an indifferent appetite.

Evening meal

Assuming that this is the smaller of the two main meals of the day, consider many of the light foods such as soups, omelettes, salads and sandwiches.

- A liquidizer in the house opens the door to all kinds of tasty home-made soups – leek and potato, mixed vegetables, tomato etc; in winter; watercress, cucumber and avocado in summer. Add a dash of cream for extra calories.
- Try to make omelettes as varied as possible but don't try to cram them full of meat, fish or vegetables or they will become too much. The same goes for sandwiches. Use very thin bread (preferably wholemeal) and cut the sandwiches very small. Egg mayonnaise is easily digested as are the variety of fish and meat pastes you can buy already made-up.

Late-night drinks

- Many people have a late-night drink to help them sleep, and people with cancer are no exception. Once again, it is a good way of getting calories either as straightforward hot milk or as cocoa, hot chocolate, Horlicks, etc. Keep a range of drinks to vary the flavour.

Supplements

Everyone is familiar with nourishing drinks such as Complan and Build Up and these are useful stand-bys for bad days or times when you have not had time to make some soup. They are available in a variety of flavours. In addition, there are two types of supplements you can add to food for people with cancer who are not eating well: high-protein and high-energy supplements. Both sorts are available on prescription. High-protein supplements, as the name suggests, allow you to boost the protein content of the diet without having to eat extra. And energy supplements are full of calories. You can add either type of supplement to anything which contains liquids. So this can be something as obvious as drinks, soups, sauces and casseroles or something less obvious such as semolina, jellies or other instant desserts.

You will have to experiment with the amount of the supplements you use before they change the taste or texture of the food. But, as an example, a teaspoon of one of the energy supplements such as Polycose or Maxijoule contains about 20 calories. Add a dessertspoonful to a mug of soup and you'll have taken in an extra 50 calories or so without thinking about it.

Dieticians explain that it is probably more important to boost the energy than the protein intake. This is because even someone who is not eating well will probably take in an adequate amount of protein. But this protein is precious. Without a sufficient calorie intake the body will start to break down the protein for energy, leading to muscle wasting. If you can keep up the calorie intake from other non-protein sources then there will be no need for the body to break down the protein which is needed for other body functions.

The normal diet contains all the vitamins necessary for good health, but someone who is not eating well may well need some extra vitamins. So it is worth checking with the doctor whether this applies to you or your relative.

*

The most important thing about all food for difficult appetites is to find out exactly what the friend or relative with cancer fancies to eat. When the answer is 'Nothing much, you choose' suggest a few options to them; often the rather negative attitude can be changed by something particularly appetizing.

Always do small portions, but make sure there is enough for second helpings. Make the food look as attractive as possible and lay it out on a big plate so it looks even smaller than it really is. Bear in mind that cooking smells may make a healthy person drool at the mouth but can be very off-putting to someone who is not feeling well. On the whole, steer clear of spicy, highly seasoned or deep-fried foods unless there is a particular request.

Many people assume that people with cancer should not drink alcohol, especially if they are taking drugs. Occasionally there are medicines which do not mix, so it is worth checking with your doctor. But on the whole a glass of sherry or wine can stimulate the appetite and possibly the spirits too. All alcohol is high in calories, particularly beers and lagers, so that is another reason to keep a few bottles to hand.

FEELING SICK

Nausea and vomiting are common side-effects of chemo-therapy, but they are not mandatory! Just as hair loss does not occur with all anti-cancer drugs, so sickness is more common with some treatments than others. Many people sail through their chemotherapy without any trouble at all. And it is impossible to predict who will feel sick as people vary so much in their responses to the same drugs.

Treatment involving combinations of drugs is more likely to cause nausea and vomiting. A variety of drugs are available to prevent sickness; as a group they are called anti-emetics. Simple measures similar to those taken by pregnant women can help reduce the risk of nausea and vomiting. Eating a dry biscuit or toast first thing in the morning, not getting out of bed too quickly and avoiding fatty or spicy foods are all useful.

Once a person's reactions to chemotherapy are established it is possible to tailor anti-emetics to their own particular needs. The drugs and the way in which they are given will depend to some extent on whether the anti-cancer drugs are being given through a drip, an injection or in tablet form. Some anti-cancer drugs, particularly the injectable ones, cause vomiting almost immediately, within minutes or hours of starting treatment. So people are given an injection of an anti-emetic at the same time as their chemotherapy to prevent or cut down vomiting, and then they are given anti-sickness tablets regularly during the next 24 hours or so to prevent nausea.

Other drugs do not cause their sickness effect for several hours and so anti-emetic tablets taken at the first signs of trouble are all that are needed. In recent years there has been a lot of interest in anti-emetics, and some much better drugs are now available than in the past.

There are no hard-and-fast rules about eating during a course of chemotherapy. Some people find they make little or no change to their diet, while others find it easier not to eat in the hours before and immediately after their treatment or they eat only small amounts. Some people who know they are prone to sickness prefer to have something in their stomach to bring up rather than to go through hours of uncomfortable retching.

Obviously, nausea and vomiting are not pleasant. But many people find that with a little thoughtful dietary planning, careful use of anti-emetics and a little extra thought and consideration from family and friends they can get through their course of chemotherapy with a minimum of stomach upset.

AVOIDING MOUTH ULCERS

Many people suffer needlessly from painful mouth ulcers when a little thought before treatment begins can prevent them. A number of anti-cancer drugs can cause mouth ulcers and the biggest culprits are methotrexate and mitomycin C.

The secret of prevention is to begin mouthwashes as soon as the mouth begins to feel sore and to keep the whole area scrupulously clean. This means regular teeth cleaning too, but use a soft tooth-brush to avoid aggravating painful gums. Commonly used mouthwashes are Oraldene and chlorhexidine in water. And for people who have already got mouth ulcers a number of an-aesthetic gels can be smeared on the inside of the mouth to reduce the pain. Once again, spicy foods are likely to aggravate them as are cigarettes and alcohol. Cool drinks and chilled yoghurts may help to soothe sore mouths and, if it is the lips which are sore and preventing you from eating, try covering them with gauze and eating from a small spoon or drinking through a straw.

If you are being treated with methotrexate there is another option – a drug called folinic acid. Methotrexate interferes with the metabolism of cancer cells and, at the same time, impairs the metabolism in cells lining the mouth. But these cells can be 'rescued' by using folinic acid about 24 hours after chemotherapy. This enables the metabolism of the mouth cells to continue normally. Once the methotrexate has passed through the body the cells in the mouth are no longer at risk and the folinic acid can be stopped. It can also be used to treat established ulcers as long as there is no infection.

WILL I LOSE MY HAIR?

Losing your hair is physically the least serious side-effect of chemotherapy but it is frequently the most devastating psy-chologically. Nausea, tiredness, bruising, even infection pale into insignificance at the first tell-tale strands of hair in your comb or on your pillow. It seems like the last straw.

Not all anti-cancer drugs cause hair loss. The chief culprits are doxorubicin (adriamycin), etoposide, cyclophosphamide, cisplatin and vincristine. So that leaves melphalan, BCNU, CCNU and methotrexate amongst the two dozen or so drugs which do not cause hair loss. The problem is that most people with cancer are given mixtures of cytotoxic drugs and if one of these causes hair loss then that is enough.

People do vary in the amount of hair which they lose and in the number of treatments before it begins to fall out. Some get away with just some thinning of the hair and it does depend on the drugs you are given. You are likely to lose eyebrows and possibly eye-lashes but not nails or teeth.

The hair will not all fall out at once but you may find it beginning to collect in your comb within a few weeks of starting treatment. On the other hand, it may take two or three cycles of treatment (if you are only having drugs every three or four weeks) for the hair to start falling out. There are also certain things you can do to reduce or slow down the hair loss:

● Cut down the frequency with which you wash your hair and use a very mild shampoo such as one of those recommended for babies.
● Avoid using a hairdrier or heated rollers: let your hair dry naturally.
● Do not use any chemicals on your hair – dyes, perms, highlights.
● Don't brush your hair harshly and use the wide-toothed side of your comb.

Anti-cancer drugs kill the hair by getting into the follicles or roots at the base of each hair-shaft. As the roots die, the hairs fall out. This is true of hair all over your body, so you won't just lose it on your scalp but on your face, under your arms and in the pubic region. Men will lose much of their body hair too.

Cooling the scalp can prevent some anti-cancer drugs getting into and killing the hair follicles. The technique, which means wearing an ice-cap at about −20 °C, is only really effective for the drug Adriamycin. If this is being used on its own the ice-cap can work very well, but if it is being used alongside other anti-cancer drugs which cause hair loss it may be of little value.

The cap has to be worn throughout the time that the drug is being given, which is why it is impractical if treatment is with daily tablets or with intravenous drips taking several hours. For Adriamycin this means 15 minutes before the injection is given and 45 minutes afterwards.

Ice-caps do not suit everyone: they are very cold and some people do find them too uncomfortable. Some hospitals make their own caps out of ice-packs and towels, others use commercial brands. Their success depends on how they are used – whether they are sufficiently cold and stay on for long enough.

Anyone who has chemotherapy with drugs known to cause hair loss is entitled to a wig on the National Health Service (NHS), though there is a charge if you are treated as an out-patient. Some people prefer not to have a wig and use a variety of hats and scarves to camouflage their hair loss. Even if you don't think you will wear a wig it is advisable to choose one when you start treatment, just in case. It is much better to choose a wig calmly when you still have your hair rather than in a mad rush when it starts to fall out. Take your time and don't feel rushed. Remember that your head will be smaller without your hair so consider an elasticated wig which will adapt according to the amount of hair you have. You may feel like a complete change in style and colour, but bear in mind that your hair will fall out slowly and you may want to blend in strands of your own hair, especially at the front and sides, to make it look more natural and this will be difficult if you are naturally dark and you have chosen a blond wig.

The most important thing to remember about hair loss from cancer chemotherapy is that your hair will grow back after you stop treatment; you will probably have a full head of hair about three to four months after treatment stops. Previous chemotherapy will make you neither more nor less likely to lose your hair next time around. And although prolonged chemotherapy may delay the return of your hair it will come back however many treatments you have.

HOW CAN I AVOID BECOMING INFERTILE?

It is difficult to gauge how commonly infertility results from chemotherapy because most people who have anti-cancer drugs are older and do not try to have children after treatment. The only real experience therefore lies with the treatment of the leukaemias, Hodgkin's disease and the cancers of the male and female reproductive organs – all of which do occur in younger people who may still want to have children.

The treatment of cancers of the ovaries and womb tends to involve surgical removal of these tissues so the question of whether chemotherapy affects fertility does not arise. And although chemotherapy does disrupt the female menstrual cycle this generally returns to normal after treatment, especially in younger women. Children born to women who have had chemotherapy are just as likely to be normal and healthy as any others. Couples are advised to use contraceptives during chemotherapy, however, because of the risk to the foetus of being exposed to these powerful drugs.

Men can become infertile after chemotherapy but this depends very much on the drugs which are used. In such cases men who may want to have children in the future should ask about sperm banking. Temporary infertility can also occur after chemotherapy and the time it takes for a sperm count to return to normal varies enormously, from six months to at least seven years. So couples not planning children are advised to use contraceptives even after the male partner has had chemotherapy.

Not everyone can produce a sperm sample suitable for banking and it isn't every hospital which has access to facilities. But if it is something which is important to you insist on finding out what is available. There is little on the NHS. Your doctor can contact the Royal College of Obstetricians and Gynaecologists for a list of artificial insemination clinics, some of which have sperm banks. The British Pregnancy Advisory Service runs sperm banks and a list of these is available from the head office (Austy Manor, Wootton Wawen, Solihull B95 6BX). Although this is probably the cheapest, non-NHS facility available it is likely to cost you about £100 to begin with and £20 a year for storage. Whichever bank you choose, allow eight weeks from approaching the bank to actually banking sperm in order for all the necessary tests and samples to be taken.

If it is your son who is to have anti-cancer drugs for leukaemia or Hodgkin's disease and he has reached puberty there is no reason why his sperm should not be banked so that he can have children as an adult.

WHAT SIDE-EFFECTS TO EXPECT FROM RADIOTHERAPY

Many people sail through their course of radiotherapy without any problems at all; in fact, if they were feeling ill before treatment they may actually start feeling better during radiotherapy. The side-effects you may experience depend very much on the part of your body which is treated. So, while in theory radiotherapy can cause nausea, tiredness, sore mouth, hair loss and 'sunburn', they are very unlikely to occur with most cancer treatments and certainly not all at once.

If you are having radiotherapy you are only likely to lose hair which is directly in the path of the rays. Thus, if you are being treated for head or neck cancers you will probably lose patches of hair on the scalp or face. If you have Hodgkin's disease or breast cancer you may be given radiotherapy to an area of the chest including the armpits, and so the hair will drop out under your arms and from your chest (if you're a man!) but not from your head. Any hair you lose during treatment will generally grow back once radiotherapy stops, but this does depend on the dose which is used.

Nausea is mainly a problem when radiotherapy is given to the abdomen. You may feel sick or actually be sick. This tends to occur mainly in the first few days of treatment, but if you find it a problem you can ask for tablets to prevent or reduce the sickness. Diarrhoea may also be a problem and this too can be relieved with drugs.

During this time you probably won't feel like eating. Don't worry if this is just for a few days; try to drink some liquids so that you don't get dehydrated and have a cup of one of the high-protein or high-calorie drinks, such as Complan or Build Up, until you are feeling better. If nausea and loss of appetite continue to be a problem try some of the tips in the section 'What to do if you can't eat' (pp. 98–103). You can lose weight very quickly when you are ill and it may not be easy to put it back. So try and tempt yourself with small, light, tasty snacks and meals at frequent intervals.

The people most likely to experience eating problems during radiotherapy are those treated for head and neck cancer. The inside of the mouth may become sore and you may have trouble swallowing. You may get mouth ulcers and your sense of taste can change. Again, milky drinks and light, soft foods which slip down easily may ease the eating problem. People are generally advised to avoid hot, spicy foods if their mouths are sore, but if you have lost your sense of taste you may prefer something with a stronger flavour. Experiment a little and see how you get on.

WILL I FEEL VERY TIRED?

Any course of treatment for cancer is likely to be physically and mentally draining. But tiredness is a common side-effect of radiotherapy. It is inevitable that some normal healthy cells will be destroyed by the treatment and that your body will be working overtime to replace them. Depending on the nature of your treatment there may be damage to the blood cells which carry oxygen around your body and while these are being replaced you are also likely to feel tired. Regular blood tests will be done to make sure that this damage from radiotherapy is kept to a minimum, but it is probably sensible to assume that you will feel more tired than usual during your treatment and so it will be necessary to plan accordingly.

It is not just physical tiredness which will take its toll. Countless people who have lain silent and alone under the vast radiotherapy machines have described how frightening it is. Surgery and chemotherapy can be pretty scary, but at least you are asleep in the operating theatre and there are always plenty of people bustling around when you are given your anti-cancer drugs. Radiotherapy is different, and medical staff may fail to warn you of the anxiety and depression you may experience during a course of treatment. And these will inevitably add to your tiredness.

So get organized before you start and ensure that your family, friends and people at work are aware that they will have to pull their weight during your treatment. Since anxiety and depression can add to fatigue make sure that you voice your fears. Take the opportunity to go and see the equipment which will be used before your treatment starts and ask as many questions as you like, however silly they may seem. Although you can't take anyone into the treatment room during your radiotherapy ask a friend or relative to go with you to the hospital at least for the first few sessions until you know how you get on with the treatment.

TAKING CARE OF YOUR SKIN

Your skin may become sensitive during radiotherapy especially if you are being treated on a delicate part of your body, such as your face or breast. It may be a bit like mild sunburn. Dusting with baby's talcum powder may soothe but if the skin is painful you can be prescribed soothing creams or lotions. Don't choose one for yourself as this may make things worse rather than better. You should avoid all deodorants, perfume and make-up on the affected area during treatment and try and keep the skin covered if you go out in the sunshine.

WILL I STILL BE ABLE TO HAVE CHILDREN?

Radiotherapy can only affect fertility if it is directed at the reproductive organs – the ovaries in women and the testes in men. It is very unlikely that radiotherapy would be given to the testes but it would be used for whole-body irradiation prior to bone marrow transplantation for leukaemia. In these circumstances any man who has reached puberty should consider whether he wants to leave sperm with a sperm bank before starting treatment.

The risks of infertility following radiotherapy are greater for women because of the position of the ovaries in the abdomen. They lie in the way, for example, if radiotherapy is planned for the abdominal lymph nodes in Hodgkin's disease. Until very recently it has been impossible to freeze and bank a woman's eggs in the same way as sperm. But children have now been born as a result of test-tube-baby techniques from eggs which were frozen and then thawed. This option will not be available routinely for some time, but in the future women who need abdominal radiotherapy may be able to bank their eggs if necessary.

AFTER SURGERY

RECOVERING FROM A MASTECTOMY

How long you need to spend in hospital after a mastectomy will depend largely on your age and fitness, but about ten days is fairly average. After the operation you will probably wake up to find a tube coming out from the dressing covering the place where your breast has been taken away. This tube drains fluid from the wound so that it heals more quickly. If you are in any pain, particularly in the first few days after the operation, you can ask for pain-killing drugs, but many women do not experience much pain after a simple mastectomy. Those who have had more extensive surgery, including removal of the lymph glands under the armpits, may get a little more pain.

The dressings will be changed regularly and the wound checked to see how it is healing. You may well be visited by a physiotherapist to help you get your arm moving on the side of your mastectomy as this may be a bit stiff, especially if your lymph glands have been removed. You will be up and about a day or two after surgery, first sitting in a chair and then walking about the ward, going to the bathroom and so on.

The drainage tube will be taken out after two or three days and the stitches after a week or so. Before you leave hospital you will be given a soft, light-weight prosthesis to slip into your bra so that your breasts match in shape and size. This is just a temporary prosthesis, called a Cumfie, and was originally designed by the Breast Care and Mastectomy Association. Because it is so soft it can be worn next to your skin while the scar is still healing.

Cumfies come in different cup sizes and you can alter the amount of filling inside them to suit your shape. You will probably wear one until your scar heals – something which varies a lot, from a couple of weeks for a fit, healthy young woman to perhaps a couple of months for a very much older lady.

Early on, you will probably be encouraged to look at and come to terms with the scar and the loss of your breast. This won't happen overnight and you should take your time. But try not to build up the first peep into a major event; the sooner you look the easier it will be, but you may prefer this to be in the privacy of your own home.

HOW TO GET THE BEST POSSIBLE PROSTHESIS FOR YOU

Once the scar has healed you will need to go back to the hospital to have your permanent prosthesis fitted. Most hospitals now have a breast prosthesis fitter attached to the hospital and she should have a range of shapes, sizes and models available to show you. There are about four major manufacturers. Most fitters do have some arrangement with one of these manufacturers and unfortunately the Breast Care and Mastectomy Association has found that some fitters tend to push the prostheses made by the manufacturer for whom they are acting as a consultant.

More women complain to the Association of problems getting a choice of prostheses than anything else – even more than those who have difficulty coming to terms with their mastectomy. If you have a mastectomy you are entitled to a prosthesis of *your* choice. Since it is only guaranteed for one year you can have a new prosthesis each year. If you are unhappy with your prosthesis you can take it back and get it exchanged. If you lose or put on weight and your prosthesis is no longer the right size you are entitled to another. Your prosthesis is going to be very important to you and you should insist on getting it right. And you should not have to buy one privately, in sheer desperation. There is nothing to show between the prostheses available on the NHS and those bought privately, except the cost; on the NHS they are totally free, privately they range from £40 to £150 – and remember that you may well need a replacement each year.

Breast prostheses come in every conceivable shape and size. There are those which simply mimic the shape of the breast itself; those with a small extension for those who have had rather more tissue removed, and those with a larger extension for women who have had tissue removed from the breast and under the arm. There are also mini-prostheses for women who have only a small part of their breast removed and simply want to build up its shape. These prostheses are made from a variety of materials but the silicone-filled models tend to be most popular as they resemble most closely the weight and feel of a woman's breast.

Manufacturers of prostheses also make bras specially designed to take the prosthesis, but most women find that ordinary bras, fitted by experts and perhaps with a pocket for the prosthesis sewn in, are perfectly satisfactory. You will only be able to get a made-to-measure NHS bra if an ordinary bra is no good. Some women find that nursing bras are especially useful, particularly in the first weeks when they feel a bit tender and are still wearing a Cumfie.

Having a breast prosthesis does not mean that you are for ever doomed to 'storm-trooper' bras, shirts buttoned to the throat and high-necked dresses. Some manufacturers design swim and beachwear specially geared to women with mastectomies, and careful placing of a few stitches or safety-pins means that even the most self-conscious can wear low-cut clothes and halter necks. Amongst its large range of useful advice leaflets the Mastectomy Association produces some helpful tips on adapting fashionable clothes to get rid of any worries you may have.

HOW WILL I FEEL ABOUT LOSING A BREAST?

There is no getting away from the fact that a mastectomy is traumatic for any woman. Just how easily and quickly you come to terms with the loss will depend a lot on the support and loving care you get from the doctors and nurses at the hospital, your family and friends. They must try to gauge how you are feeling and respond accordingly. Jollying you along and pretending not to notice the large dressing where your breast should have been may be right for some women but wrong for many others. Feel free to snap at surgeons who look extremely pleased with themselves while examining their handiwork and tell you that you're going to have a beautiful scar!

Don't be surprised that you feel depressed after your operation. Allow yourself to share your grief with other people; don't save all the tears for when you are alone. Watch out that you don't overdo things in the first few weeks after you leave hospital. You may feel very well and want to get back to normal as quickly as possible but, if you rush things, not only will you tire yourself and possibly add to any depression you may experience, you also won't have time to take stock and do your grieving. You may then suffer a delayed reaction to your mastectomy.

Recent research has shown that up to a quarter of women do suffer so much mental anguish that they need medical help. Some health authorities have started employing specialist nurses to monitor the physical and mental well-being of people with cancer and they refer women who are having trouble coping after a mastectomy for specialist help.

As already mentioned, all women will be encouraged to look at their scar as soon as possible after their mastectomy. Quite naturally, many worry about the reactions of their husbands or partners to the sight of their breast. The experience of the Breast Care and Mastectomy Association is that much of this worry is unnecessary. Just as many people with colostomies are unduly worried about what their partners will think and the same is true of women who have a mastectomy. There are no easy answers either for women who ask how to tell new partners about their mastectomy. Reactions will clearly depend very much on the strength of the relationship.

This is not to ignore the importance of a woman's image of herself. Some women decide that a prosthesis is not the answer for them and they ask for their breast to be reconstructed. A number of operations are performed and, although cosmetic surgery for women would normally have to be paid for privately, a breast reconstruction should be paid for by the NHS for someone who has had a mastectomy. So insist that you are referred to a surgeon who specializes in this type of surgery on the NHS to find out if you are a suitable candidate.

A silicone implant is generally used to build up the breast and in some operations skin is grafted from elsewhere on the body to cover the implant. Alternatively, a temporary bag can be implanted under the remaining chest tissue and slowly pumped up with liquid, like a beach-ball. Over a period of weeks the skin is slowly stretched sufficiently for the bag to be removed and the permanent implant to be inserted. This operation has the advantage that the skin over the reconstructed breast will match perfectly that on the other breast.

None of these operations is painless and without problems. It is important to discuss both the advantages and the drawbacks of the various alternatives with the surgeon before embarking on reconstructive surgery and to hear about the failed operations as well as the successes.

STOMA CARE

In some cases of bowel cancer it is not possible simply to remove the tumour and rejoin the remaining pieces of intestine.

The tumour may be at a tricky bend or too low down in the bowel – near the rectum – for the pieces of intestine to be successfully rejoined. In these cases it is necessary to bring the cut-end of the bowel to the surface of the abdomen so that waste products can be excreted. The opening which is made by bringing out the cut-end of the bowel and stitching it to the surface of the abdomen is called a stoma. It is roughly round and about the size of a 10p coin.

The name of the operation depends on the point at which the bowel is cut and brought to the surface. Thus when the stoma is created from the cut-end of the small intestine the operation is called an ileostomy and when the operation is performed further down in the colon, or large bowel, it is called a colostomy.

A stoma has neither the muscle nor nervous control over excretion of waste products which we expect from the rectum. Faecal material is excreted as and when food has been digested and it is not possible simply to store waste in the bowel until you are ready to go to the toilet. It is therefore generally necessary to wear a bag over the stoma to collect waste material.

The position of the stoma is important and you should discuss this with the surgeon and the stoma nurse before the operation. Its exact position depends in part on you. If you have rather a large 'spare tyre' below your waist it may be best to site the stoma above the flabby part, just below the waist-line, to make it easy to change the stoma bag, otherwise you will be groping around below the bulge. On the other hand, if you wear clothes with low waist-bands, on your hips, it is probably best to put the stoma lower so that the bag does not lie above the waist-band; this is especially important for men since trousers tend to be low rather than high-waisted.

Most women prefer to wear looser clothes after their colostomy or ileostomy, though there is no reason why they should not continue to wear some things which are figure hugging. The only problem is that people who are prone to wind may find that their stoma bag expands and sticks out if clothes are really skin-tight. So gathered skirts and skirts with pleating into the waist-line tend to be more popular than A-line skirts. This said, there is no reason why you should not be able to swim or sunbathe. Either you can wear a fashionable one-piece costume or you can wear a bikini with the bottom half having a high waist, or wear shorts with a bikini top. It is perfectly easy to swim while wearing a bag, though you will probably want to ensure that it is empty so that it lies flat. There is no more reason for the adhesive to come loose in water than on land.

When you are still in hospital a stoma or specialist nurse will come and explain how to look after your colostomy on a day-to-day basis. Once you are home she will continue to visit and ensure that all is progressing well and she will always be available for help if problems do arise.

There is an enormous variety of stoma bags available for people who have had colostomies or ileostomies. All are available on the NHS and if you have a stoma of any kind you are exempt from all prescription charges; that means for the stoma bags and for all drugs, whether or not they have anything to do with the stoma. Simply ask for a prescription charge exemption form from the hospital, G P's surgery or social services department and get your doctor to sign it.

The bags fall into two main groups – one-piece and two-piece appliances. The one-piece bags stick straight onto the skin around the stoma. You will need to cut a hole in the sticky backing of the bag to the correct size for your stoma, since everyone's varies. Most people are quite happy with these bags: the adhesive is strong and there is no risk of the bag coming off unless you pull it off to change it. However, some people find that the adhesive irritates the skin – this is especially common in older people and so they prefer a two-piece bag. A thin 'wafer' of flexible material with a non-irritant adhesive backing sticks onto the stoma and remains in position for three or four days. A bag is then either stuck or clipped to the 'wafer' and changed whenever necessary. This approach simply removes the need to pull adhesive away from the skin each time the bag needs to be changed.

Although the adhesive is 100 per cent effective and the risk of accident tiny, some people prefer the added security of wearing a belt around their waist to which the bag is clipped. The bag does not simply hang loose – it is still stuck to the stoma – but the belt just gives that extra degree of confidence. Many stoma bags have in-built odour filters to reduce the risk of smells.

There are no hard and fast rules about how often you will

need to change the bag. Many people get into a routine, so that although they still have no control over when something passes out of their stoma it tends to happen at particular times of day. Sometimes it is possible to feel material coming out, sometimes not. The bag may only need changing once a day, or it may be more: that will depend partly on your diet and partly on your reactions to it – whether you prefer to change it the moment material has been passed or whether you prefer to wait until the bag has filled up. Disposal of bags is quite straightforward: the bag is filled with water and the bottom-end clipped off so that the contents can be emptied into the toilet. The empty bag can then be wrapped in newspaper or some other bag and put in with the ordinary household waste. Refuse collectors do not have X-ray eyes and there are far worse things in other people's rubbish!

People tend to assume that once you have a colostomy or ileostomy you will have to give up all your favourite foods for ever – either because they are too rich and likely to cause constipation, too spicy and likely to cause diarrhoea or too fibrous and likely to cause wind. This is simply not true and the best advice is to try out different foods and see what effect they have. Ideally, you should aim to eat a diet which gives faecal material which is easy to pass through the stoma. Too hard and it will be painful, too soft and you will get diarrhoea.

The place where the bowel has been cut will also affect the composition of the faeces. The higher up the operation the less digested the food and consequently the looser the bowel movement. Thus someone with an ileostomy is likely to pass rather loose, fluid stools whereas someone with a colostomy low down in the bowel will pass a stool little different from that of someone with an intact bowel.

As well as diet, other agents are available to harden or soften faecal material for people experiencing problems. Methylcellulose is commonly used to treat constipation or diarrhoea. The granules are dissolved in water and the amount of fluid varied according to whether you are trying to harden and bind the stool together because of diarrhoea or soften it because of constipation.

More recently, a growing number of people have started using an alternative to stoma bags, called irrigation. Literally, this involves washing out the intestine of faecal content. It has the advantage in that once established it only has to be done on average once every 48 hours; it removes the need for stoma bags and a simple stoma cap is all that is needed to cover the stoma; there is no risk of smells or wind. On the debit side, the procedure does take about an hour and some people find the idea of washing out their intestine distasteful. A tube is inserted into the stoma and water carefully and slowly poured into the intestine; once in the tube is then attached to a disposal tube leading out into the toilet.

If you are considering trying irrigation it is very important first to speak to your consultant as some stomas are not suitable for irrigation. It is also important to arrange for a demonstration from your stoma nurse before trying it out for yourself, and the equipment should be prescribed by your doctor. Don't experiment on your own! Swapping to irrigation does not have to be permanent; if you wish you can use the method during the summer, say, when you don't want to be fussing with bags under light summer clothing, and return to stoma bags during the winter when you may find sitting in the bathroom naked from the waist down for an hour every two days rather chilly.

One of the commonest questions people ask before and after a colostomy or ileostomy is 'How will it affect my sex life?' Most people are worried that their partners will take one look at it and run screaming from the room! In the experience of the Colostomy Welfare Group, a society which provides advice and support to thousands of people who have had the operation, the whole problem is much overrated! It is generally the person with the colostomy who is most worried and finds it hardest to believe the partner who insists that it really does not matter. It is the partner who takes it in his or her stride. The approach you take depends very much on your own particular relationship. Some people like their partner to see the stoma and at least know what it looks like. During sex, some people wear a stoma bag, checking first that it is empty, and some like to cover it by putting it in a small cotton pouch; these are widely available. Alternatively, if you know that you are making love at a time of day when it is very unlikely that anything will come out of the stoma you may prefer simply to cover it with a stoma cap or with a light dressing or piece of gauze. Take things in your stride; don't feel that you must face the situation the moment you leave hospital, but don't let it build up into a major issue by avoiding sex with your partner month after month.

Some people also worry about coping with their stoma when they are abroad. Again, there is no need to worry. Make sure that you pack plenty of spare bags. Within reason, there is no official limit on the number of stoma bags which a GP may prescribe at one visit. Stoma bags, of course, are available abroad. Europeans, Americans, Asians and Australians all have colostomies and ileostomies too! But they may have different brand names and you will have to pay for them, except in Europe provided you get a form E111 for medical supplies in EEC countries. When travelling, particularly to countries with less than perfect sanitary arrangements, you may find it worthwhile taking supplies of anti-diarrhoea pills and laxatives to cope with any digestive problems which may arise.

People with ileostomies and colostomies do not become social pariahs. You can tell as many or as few people as you like about your operation. And remember that they won't be aware that you have a stoma bag unless you tell them. So don't feel self-conscious!

AFTER A LARYNGECTOMY

Some 700 laryngectomy operations are performed each year. Caught early, the outlook for people with laryngeal cancer is very good and it is thought that at least 4000 people in the UK are coping with everyday life without a voice-box. In North America, where the operation is more often done as first-line treatment in preference to radiotherapy, thousands more people have learned to communicate without a larynx.

The larynx, as well as carrying the vocal cords which make sound, is also an important part of the respiratory system. Once it is gone air can no longer pass through your mouth and nose down to your lungs so an alternative opening has to be made in the neck to enable air to reach the lungs. This opening is a stoma and is called a tracheostomy.

Depending on the tissue in your stoma you will either be

given a short piece of tubing which protrudes from the stoma, or not. The tissue in some people's laryngectomies is prone to closing up; it does not happen overnight, but putting a tracheostomy tube into the stoma prevents this from happening and you needing an operation to dilate the stoma. So if you are given a tube to put into the stoma you should wear it at all times.

People with stomas in their necks are also advised to keep the stoma covered with the stoma cap. This does not stop air from getting in but it does prevent dust and dirt from irritating the stoma and possibly causing an infection.

During the operation to remove the larynx a feeding tube will be passed up your nose and down into your stomach to enable you to receive a liquid diet while the area around the larynx heals. Although the tube which carries food, the oesophagus, is separate from the air-carrying trachea, the two tubes lie alongside one another and the movement of normal solid food being swallowed and passing down the oesophagus would disrupt healing in the trachea. The naso-gastric tube which is therefore inserted is usually left in place for about ten days.

When the first few days after the operation are over you will be visited by a speech therapist. He or she will teach you how to communicate without a voice-box. The aim is to teach you how to speak with air from your oesophagus rather than the trachea. You will learn how to take air in through your mouth and make it go down the oesophagus. This air is then brought up again into the mouth and used to make a sound. Individual words are framed by the movement of your tongue and mouth, as normal. The process of taking in and bringing up air is similar to burping, but instead of the single-tone noise of the burp you use the air to make words. It is called oesophageal speech.

It is relatively easy to describe the process on paper, but oesophageal speech is not easy and some people do not learn how to do it. For them, one alternative is a speech-aid. These are small hand-held devices about the size of a telephone bleep which produce a single-tone sound. The device is held against the face and the words shaped by the muscles in your mouth are projected by the tone as speech. This is not ideal and the speech does tend to sound rather robotic. But if you have had trouble learning oesophageal speech a speech-aid does at least enable you to communicate verbally. Speech-aids vary in complexity and price and it is best to go for the one which suits you, regardless of cost. Some people prefer the simplest, cheapest devices, others do better with the more complex ones. Either way, they are available on the NHS through the hospital at which you are treated. You may have to persevere to get the device you want, but you are entitled to it.

Various experimental operations are being performed to enable people to speak more easily after a laryngectomy and so avoid the need for oesophageal speech and it is worth asking what is available. A small but growing number of hospitals are using valves inserted into the neck to control the passage of air up from the lungs. It goes in through the stoma and down to the lungs. But instead of coming back out of the stoma it is diverted upwards into the mouth so that words can be shaped normally. This method is by no means perfect and problems can arise, but it seems likely that developments of this operation will be the way forward for laryngectomies of the future.

Anyone who has had a laryngectomy is exempt from prescription charges for all medicines whether related to their operation or not. Simply get your GP or consultant to sign a prescription exemption form available at the hospital, surgery or social services department. People with laryngectomies do have to be careful to avoid respiratory infections since these tend to be more serious. Fluid and mucus can build up in the respiratory passages and be difficult to get rid of without a tracheostomy tube.

Various cards and discs are available for people to carry about with them warning that resuscitation needs to be carried out via the stoma in the event of someone who has had a laryngectomy not being able to breathe on their own. Mouth-to-mouth artificial respiration must be replaced with mouth-to-stoma.

Removal of the larynx is a terrifying prospect for those of us used to speaking normally. Communication for someone who has had a laryngectomy can be difficult and frustrating. A positive approach is very important right from the start to avoid sinking into a silent world. Close friends and relatives will learn to lip read, but strangers won't. The onus is on the laryngectomee to adapt and overcome the difficulties.

YOU'LL STILL BE A WOMAN AFTER A HYSTERECTOMY

Many women, faced with the news that they need to have their womb and possibly their ovaries removed, believe that they are about to lose their sexuality. They know that they must forfeit the chance of getting pregnant but they assume that with that will go their figure, their looks and their interest in sex. They know that the menopause is a difficult time for any woman and can see only the unfairness of getting hot flushes, depression and vaginal dryness ten or twenty years before their time. They cause themselves a lot of unnecessary heartache.

The most common misconception about hysterectomy is that you will automatically go through the menopause. If you have your womb removed you will stop having periods because there is no womb lining left to come away each month. But it is your ovaries which produce the oestrogen and the eggs and these will go on working. Wherever possible, surgeons do leave behind the ovaries when they do a hysterectomy because they are well aware of the importance of oestrogen to women who are not yet of menopausal age.

Provided that the cancer is limited to the womb or cervix there should be no need to take away the ovaries. If the cancer has started in the ovaries then it is virtually impossible to save them from surgery. But if only one ovary is affected and a woman particularly wants to remain fertile it may be possible just to remove the cancerous ovary and leave the other one and the womb intact. In such cases it is important to weigh up the risks to your life if minute amounts of tumour, as yet invisible to the surgeon, have spread, against your desire for children.

If you have a hysterectomy, whether or not your ovaries are removed at the same time, you will have to spend about ten days to two weeks in hospital. The operation will be done under general anaesthetic and when you come round you will have a drainage tube coming out of your abdomen and probably a fluid drip going into your arm. The drainage tube is there to get rid of excess fluid from your wound so that it will heal more quickly. The drip is put up to replace fluids from your body since you will be unable to drink normally immediately after your operation.

Sometimes there will also be a tube draining water from your bladder. This tube, called a catheter, will have been put into your water passage, the urethra, during the operation. You will probably feel some pain after your operation, but that can easily be relieved by drugs. If you are still uncomfortable be sure to tell the nurses so that you can be given more pain-killers.

All of the tubes will be removed within the first few days of your operation and you will be encouraged to get up and about as soon as possible. A hysterectomy is a major operation and just how quickly you recover will depend on your age and general health. A physiotherapist will probably come and give you breathing and other exercises to do while you are in bed.

The stitches will be removed as soon as the wound in your abdomen is healed. You will be left with a narrow scar, either horizontal or perpendicular, low on your abdomen and this will fade to a fine line as the months pass. Once your stitches are out you will be able to go home, but you should take things very gently at first. You will probably need about two months off work, and leave the housework to someone else! Everyone's recovery is different so take things at your own pace.

You are only likely to get menopausal symptoms if you have had both ovaries removed and even then it is not mandatory! If you do get symptoms – hot flushes, dryness in the vagina and pain during sexual intercourse or you are worried or upset – be sure to go and see your GP or find out if there is a menopause clinic at a nearby hospital to which you can be referred.

After a hysterectomy you will be advised not to make love for about six weeks until you have had a chance to heal inside. Initially you may be rather sore and some lubricant jelly from the chemist will probably help. If you have had your ovaries removed and simply using KY jelly is not enough, or you are getting other menopausal symptoms which are unacceptable to you, ask about having hormone replacement therapy (HRT). This is exactly what it sounds like. You will be given hormones very similar to those you are no longer producing. These can be taken as tablets, or increasingly popular are the 'depot' injections. These involve injecting a larger amount of hormone in the form of a tiny pellet or capsule which releases the hormone over several months. Before you start HRT you will need a physical check-up and your blood pressure measured. Not everyone is suitable for treatment and doctors may recommend delaying the start of treatment until they are sure there is no sign of a recurrence of the cancer.

HRT does not mean that you will start having periods again – that is not possible if your womb has been removed – but it does mean that you will avoid both the short-term upset of menopausal symptoms and the long-term risk of fragile bones, osteoporosis, which affects many elderly women.

If you do decide to have HRT after your womb and ovaries have been removed there is no real time-limit on how long this can continue. You will need regular check-ups and you may decide periodically to stop treatment to see if menopausal symptoms recur. But there is no need to suffer in silence after a hysterectomy even if your ovaries have been removed as well.

Chapter Seven

GETTING SUPPORT

'. . . the medical services were excellent, but there was a desperate need for someone to listen when I needed to get things off my chest . . .' (Petra Griffiths, co-founder of CancerLink).

'I was in tears every morning when I found hairs all over the bed. Then I hit on the solution of a hairnet . . . such a small thing I wished I'd known at the beginning . . .' (Dr Vicky Clement-Jones, founder of the British Association of Cancer United Patients)

Many people are devastated when they first learn they have cancer. Some describe the diagnosis as like an explosion going off in the head – you hear the words but cannot take in their meaning. Others talk of being catapulted into a strange world or hurtling down a chute. Partners and relatives are sometimes so shocked that they are surprised the outside world is still going on as normal. Ethel Helman describes this feeling very vividly in *An Autumn Life* (Faber and Faber 1986), an account of her surgeon husband's last illness. Looking from the window of the ward where he was being treated for cancer of the colon she wondered how it was possible that everything looked the same. 'Why hadn't the traffic drawn to a halt?' she wondered. 'Why hadn't the sun stopped shining?' And, finally, 'How was it possible that everyone could not see how much I was suffering?'

This cry of the heart surely echoes the feelings of most of those touched by cancer. The disease has powerful, fearful associations, from which few of us are immune, whatever our background, training, or professional insight. Cancer *is* frightening for doctors, nurses, friends, families, as well as for those who have it. And intense feelings of anger, loss, fear and depression on diagnosis are not a sign of inadequacy or instability. They are normal.

Some people do deal with cancer rather as they might face a diseased appendix or an annoying verruca – something to be taken out and forgotten as soon as possible. But for many the process is drawn out and nothing like as simple as that. So looking for support, early on, is a sensible response, not a sign of ineptitude.

WHY ME?

Nobody feels ready to face cancer. How could they?

The previously successful feel that they have been unfairly tripped up, the unfulfilled take it as further evidence they were never meant to get a crack at life, the young are stunned at having mortality brought home to them; and the elderly must face up to leaving behind relationships developed over decades.

Parents worry about the future of their offspring just as the childless mourn for the children they may now never have. There is no right time to learn your life is threatened. Very rarely can the experience of cancer be easily or quickly assimilated.

Looking for reasons why or possible explanations is a natural way of coming to terms with any very upsetting experience. But nobody knows what causes the majority of cancers. And in the absence of any scientific explanation it is very common for people to look to their own past for possible causes. Counsellors in this field find that people whose cancer has just been diagnosed often fill the whole of the first interview going back over what has happened up to that point in their lives.

Some people can only come to terms with their illness by placing it in context of what went before. And this may involve a period of withdrawal or intense introspection when the person tries to answer 'Why me?' to their satisfaction. This, of course, is impossible on any reasonable basis. But that is not to say that no one finds meaning in serious illness. Far from it. Very many personal accounts from people with cancer speak about the 'secondary gains' that the experience often brings: sharpened values, a heightened appreciation of life and a greater sense of what really matters.

But for the first few weeks following diagnosis disbelief, anger, resentment and a sense of 'unfairness' often prevail. These feelings are a normal part of unravelling the experience and gradually coming to terms with your changed world. But knowing your feelings are normal is no consolation when your mind is going round and round, unable to find rest. Some people find it helpful to remind themselves that they have coped with other crises and so will cope with this, bewildering and senseless as it seems. One woman who was very anxious after an operation used to say to herself 'This is a mystery' whenever she felt herself worrying and found that that quietened her mind. It is also a step towards accepting the uncertainty cancer involves.

On a more practical level an engrossing book, soothing music in your personal stereo headset or knitting can ease the tension of out-patients clinics or the tedium of ward life. (That is less obvious than it sounds, judging by the number of worried, empty-handed people you see in hospital waiting areas.)

Studies have shown that more than 50 per cent of people with cancer suffer depression. And in the case of women who have undergone a mastectomy this is frequently severe enough to require psychiatric help. One study of psychiatric problems in the year after mastectomy showed that 39 per cent of women experienced serious anxiety, depression or sexual difficulties.

Yet rather than seek support, people with cancer often draw into themselves in the belief that they should, or must, cope alone. Many become isolated from the very supports they would normally rely on in time of adversity, partly out of sensitivity to others' reactions: 'I don't want to embarrass my friends by saying I've got cancer or talking about the nasty effects of treatment' and 'They don't seem to know what to ask me because they're frightened of what I'll tell them' are common remarks by people who have distanced themselves from friends. Such comments are not unrealistic – people often are unsure and slightly wary about communicating with people who have cancer. But all the more reason for making sure you get support from somewhere. Isolation will only make you more vulnerable to depression.

Realizing that depression, anxiety and sexual problems often go unrecognized in hospitals – either because people do not voice their difficulties or doctors fail to pick them up – many cancer departments are trying to build in some form of support. Several hospitals have specialist nurses/counsellors to talk to patients at length, before, during and after their hospital stay so that anxieties and problems with adaptation can be helped from the start. There are some 300 stoma and 40 breast-care specialist nurses working in hospitals. Some make a point of visiting people in their homes before they come into hospital to help with practical difficulties, such as finding someone to care for the children, as well as worries about the illness itself.

Specialist nurses offer people with cancer a chance to talk over their feelings and difficulties at all stages of the illness and treatment, from diagnosis onwards. Some sit in with the doctor when the diagnosis is given. They can prove a very valuable link for people worried about recurrences by keeping in touch after the person has returned home from hospital. Besides offering advice on side-effects, prostheses and communication difficulties they give people a chance to 'work through' their anger at having cancer and so prevent them becoming stuck in depression. They give one-to-one interviews, lasting about an hour in the first instance, and often involve partners. Where they see more specialist support is needed, such as psychiatric consultation or psychosexual counselling, they can advise on where to go.

HOSPITAL SOCIAL WORKERS

Social workers generally come to public attention only when one of their number has failed to prevent a child death which everyone, in retrospect, judges perfectly preventable. Few people think of consulting one before they run into problems or sense the need for someone to mediate on their behalf with the authorities. But in the hospital setting they can sometimes give patients and families a welcome sense of continuity as well as practical advice and emotional support.

Social workers advise on Department of Health and Social Security (DHSS) benefits such as fares payments, grants, transport and dealing with bills and debts. They can also write letters on a client's behalf to the telephone, gas and electric authorities and the building society, if need be.

When someone is returning home after in-patient treatment the social worker can contact local community nursing staff and social services to arrange home care, meals on wheels and home helps. Where children need to be looked after, because a parent or sibling is in hospital, the social worker should be able to make arrangements through the social services department. Where a child is going back to school after cancer treatment the social worker often contacts the school first, and sometimes talks to the class, clearing up misconceptions about cancer being catching and explaining any changes in the child's appearance. Hospital social workers often remain in touch with people with cancer and their families for several years after the initial hospital stay. People who are especially worried about a recurrence may find it helpful to keep in contact in this way.

Nobody can take in all the implications of their illness immediately, nor, realistically, can they expect their hospital appointments to provide all the information they find they need. Several studies have shown that people forget up to half of what they are told in consultations and they frequently come away having forgotten the one question they wanted to ask. Besides, some people feel happier unburdening themselves and their fears anonymously to someone at the end of a telephone, rather than in a face-to-face interview with someone they see regularly.

ORGANIZATIONS WITH USEFUL INFORMATION

Telephone cancer information services offer time, the possibility of unhurried explanations (calls sometimes last twenty minutes or more) and an opportunity to ring back again and again if need be. While some people need to ring only once for a specific piece of information others phone regularly and often speak to the same person (who has built up a picture of their situation).

BACUP (British Association of Cancer United Patients and their families and friends)

Launched in 1985 by Dr Vicky Clement-Jones as a result of her experience with ovarian cancer, BACUP provides telephone information and advice on all aspects of cancer, and is staffed by nurses who have more than thirty years' experience of cancer nursing. They in turn are backed up by a large medical and scientific advisory panel. More than three-quarters of the callers are women, with breast cancer accounting for about a third of all queries. Staff are happy to give detailed explanations of treatments and possible side-effects and to provide emotional support for those distressed by cancer. They are used to people ringing up when they are upset and unsure what to do and appreciate that people with cancer often need to be given information several times before understanding it. The staff do not recommend specific treatments but will outline the options and help clarify the questions to be put to the appropriate doctor.

They can also put callers in touch with local groups and counsellors. BACUP aims to provide detailed practical advice on sources of financial help, home nursing, screening, wigs and prostheses, legal problems and research centres. The nurses answering the telephone have access to cancer experts and the service is evaluated by means of questionnaires.

BACUP produces a newspaper and leaflets on diet, hair care, Hodgkin's disease and cancer of the ovary, bladder, breast, cervix, colon and rectum, kidney, lungs, oesophagus, pancreas, prostate, skin, stomach, testes, thyroid and uterus. Personal callers are welcome. Aimed at improving all aspects of life for the person with cancer the service welcomes input from callers, whether tips on wig care, the name of a sympathetic insurance broker, a dish which has proved successful for those with diet problems, or a new source of financial help for people unable to work because of their illness.

CANCERLINK

'My father has been told he must have radiotherapy. Will his hair fall out?'

'What's the latest treatment for cancer of the cervix?'

'I don't think they're doing enough for her up at the hospital. But I don't know what to ask.'

'Where can I find out about home nursing?'

'I've tried the Bristol Diet but find it difficult. Does it really help?'

'How can you tell when someone is dying? What does it look like?'

From their offices in North London the two nurses running CancerLink's information service attempt to answer up to forty such calls a day, their work-load rising and falling in line with media coverage of cancer. They do not promote any particular therapy to callers but attempt to clarify what has already been said about the individual's illness and to provide appropriate help, whether in the form of practical information or general reassurance.

CancerLink was set up in May 1982 by four people with personal or professional interests in cancer: health writer Petra Griffiths, who had been successfully treated for Hodgkin's disease in 1981; Anne Jenkinson, an immunologist at the Imperial Cancer Research Fund, who had been successfully treated for choriocarcinoma; Val Box, Cancer Education Adviser for the South West Regional Cancer Organization; and Julian Gross, head of the Department of Cell Differentiation at the Imperial Cancer Research Fund. They felt there was a need for an information service on all aspects of cancer including details of practical and emotional support (groups, home nursing services, day centres, welfare benefits).

The following year a support groups service was started, with training courses for those wishing to set up new groups. Refresher courses to improve the knowledge and communication skills of those in established groups are run about every three months.

An analysis of CancerLink's calls showed almost 40 per cent were from people with cancer, some 12 per cent from partners and most of the remainder from family and friends. Questions on treatment were most frequently followed by those on the disease itself, home and practical care, eating problems, what to tell children, screening, getting a second opinion, asking about the prognosis and sexual problems.

CancerLink also keeps a list of pain clinics in Britain and

Ireland, including the names of doctors to contact. The nurses running the information service have found that most GPs are happy to refer people for specialist opinion on pain control, when their own efforts are not proving effective.

As well as its own network of self-help groups (see Chapter 8 on groups), CancerLink maintains the *Directory of Cancer Support Groups in the UK* listing more than 100 organizations. Guidelines and training courses are available for people interested in running a group.

CancerLink also publishes a *Directory of Useful Organizations* covering those giving help to people with specific types of cancer, such as the Leukaemia Care Society and the Urostomy Association, as well as sources of help for nursing care, hospice information, practical and financial assistance, the elderly and disabled, sexuality and cancer, counselling and complementary methods of care.

OTHER ORGANIZATIONS

CALL (Cancer Aid and Listening Line) was established in Manchester in 1983 by Tom Brown, following his recovery from Hodgkin's disease. The telephone lines are staffed by volunteers, trained by Dr Peter Maguire, a psychiatrist, who has made extensive studies of communication in cancer. The volunteers offer support and information on available services. No medical advice is given.

Cancercare Lancaster, set up in 1984 at the Royal Lancaster Infirmary, provides a support group and telephone information service for people in North Lancashire and South Cumbria, and a Quarterly newspaper, *Rapport*. The information line is staffed by volunteers and professionals.

The *Mastectomy Association* answers some 1700 telephone and postal inquiries a month, many on bras and prostheses. The Association has some 1600 volunteer helpers throughout Britain – women who have undergone mastectomy or lumpectomy and are willing to visit or advise others, before and after their operation. The Association tries to match up women in terms of age and location. Free leaflets are available on bras, prostheses, swimwear, living with the loss of a breast, breast biopsy and mastectomy, as well as a list of stockists.

The *Colostomy Welfare Group* (CWG) answers more than 8000 queries a year and welcomes personal callers as well as running a telephone and postal advice service. Detailed medical queries are normally referred to a specialist nurse but the CWG can advise on after-care, rehabilitation and psychological difficulties. It also has more than 100 volunteers who have colostomies and are willing to visit others. Leaflets include: *To the Patient about to have a Colostomy*; *To the Patient with a Colostomy*; *Appliance Handbook*; *Thoughtful Eating*; *Wind, Constipation and Diarrhoea*; *Travel Advice*; *Irrigation*; and *Convalescent Homes*. The CWG also provides information on appliance manufacturers.

The *National Association of Laryngectomee Clubs* is in touch with some 3800 people through its chain of more than 50 clubs, meeting in hospitals, throughout the British Isles and Southern Ireland. It provides a telephone information service and leaflets on such topics as stoma care and making stoma covers; also emergency cards for people who have undergone laryngectomies, explaining that they will not respond to mouth-to-mouth resuscitation. The Association can arrange, in conjunction with the local speech therapist, pre- and post-operative visits from someone who has had a laryngectomy. A newsletter, *Clan*, is produced quarterly.

Help for Health, a patient information service based at Southampton General Hospital, has details of cancer support groups in Hampshire, Dorset, Wiltshire and the Isle of Wight, as well as national associations, and a list of books written by people with cancer.

The *Women's National Cancer Control Campaign*, aimed at the early detection of breast and cervical cancer, produces leaflets on breast self-examination, smear tests and breast and cervical cancer.

The *Tenovus Cancer Information Centre*, Cardiff, keeps details of support groups in the UK and produces leaflets on cervical cytology, breast self-examination, mastectomy and answers to questions commonly asked.

The *Leukaemia Research Fund* has more than 200 branches in Britain. It produces a quarterly newsletter and leaflets on the disease in adults and children; bone marrow transplantation; Hodgkin's disease; treatment and care of childhood leukaemia and coping with childhood leukaemia in the family.

HELPING YOURSELF – THE RIGHT MENTAL ATTITUDE

*

Petra Griffiths was 32 when she was found to have Hodgkin's disease.

'I had been feeling tired for about a year which I thought was because I was doing two kinds of work. I was writing a report on patients' rights for the National Consumer Council and also teaching massage. But then I developed a cough which felt quite deep in my chest. My GP sent me for an X-ray and I was in hospital quite a few weeks . . . They finally discovered what it was by removing a tiny lump in one of the lymph glands and until I was actually told I didn't suspect at all.

'I was very shocked and very frightened at the thought of cancer as an alien thing which takes you over. I felt very powerless as if this thing was bigger than me. For a few days I wanted to cry a lot even though I was told there was a very good treatment for Hodgkin's disease. It takes quite a while to adjust.

'I read Simonton's *Getting Well Again* and found it very helpful. It helped me shift from that sense of being small and cancer taking me over. I realized I had a role to play by taking a positive attitude to my treatment. The doctors were excellent about giving information but there seemed to be a block about any forms of help coming from outside the hospital.

'At each stage the doctors were quite prepared to discuss why a particular treatment was necessary, and what might happen if I didn't have it. Previously my sympathies lay very much with the alternative side.

'When I thought of not having treatment the consultant said nobody had ever got better from Hodgkin's disease without treatment. He said that if I went away to do alternative stuff and then came back in six months there was a risk it would be much worse and more difficult to treat. So after a lot of angst I decided to have my spleen removed and start chemotherapy.

'The treatment certainly made me feel much iller than the illness, and quite weird at times. But I managed to keep working half-time and that was very helpful.

'The treatment made me debilitated and I got very depressed. But I was lucky because the people I lived with were always willing to talk. I didn't fear I wouldn't get better, it was just coping with debility and depression that was difficult. I remember feeling quite suicidal but there was always someone there.

'I had to force myself into activity at times and felt better when I did. I more or less disregarded how I felt. A lot of people in the house had flu once and I remember having to force myself to go out and meet people even though I was feeling quite strange and miles away. Sometimes if you can just pretend you feel normal it can work . . .

'Now five years on, having had cancer doesn't preoccupy me. But it is always sort of there.'

The link between positive thinking and survival has yet to be fully established. One, much quoted study conducted at King's College Hospital, London, *did* show that women with breast cancer who approached the disease with a fighting spirit had significantly higher survival rates than those who showed stoical acceptance or hopelessness. But it was a small study (57 women) whose findings need to be reproduced on a wider scale before being generally accepted. Most doctors treating people with cancer can think of many examples where spirited defiance and determination certainly seemed to prolong an individual's life. But they often add that they have seen an equal number of cases where, sadly, a hugely positive, fighting attitude has made no difference.

But nobody would disagree that a positive attitude enhances anyone's life, whether or not they have cancer. Most difficulties seem less insurmountable once they are faced in a positive way. Yet people with cancer often fail to realize that they can take control of their own attitude to treatment, if not the disease itself. A positive approach will almost certainly make you feel better in yourself whatever the cancer may be doing.

However good the information and support you obtain from hospital staff, people coming to terms with an illness, or facing some permanent change in their body, often have a strong desire to meet someone who has 'been there' and is now going on with life. If this applies to you, tell your doctor, a social worker or specialist nurse who may be able to put you in touch with someone helpful, or contact the relevant specialist association. Some hospitals have formal arrangements with local mastectomy groups to visit patients undergoing breast removal. But these are still the exceptions and usually it is up to the patient to arrange such contacts for themselves.

Talking to someone in a similar position may not appeal to everybody but is worth considering. You may feel more relaxed and able to talk about your anxieties with someone who knows the position from the inside rather than the professionals. And for their part someone who has been there can empathize and may provide valuable guidance on aspects you had not thought of. And, most important of all perhaps, they provide proof of real life after cancer, which can be very reassuring for those adjusting to a new self.

COUNSELLING – TIME FOR YOURSELF

Counselling is rather like a good friendship – hard to analyse but valuable at times of difficulty, uncertainty and unwelcome change. There is no generally agreed definition of counselling but one of its aims is to help you through bumpy times – bereavement, divorce, redundancy, illness and discord. It is also used to help people with a general feeling of malaise, lack of fulfilment or inadequacy.

Counsellors are practised listeners who try to clarify what is going on in a person's life and to help them find their own solution. The counsellor is both sounding-board and mirror – offering the client the opportunity to try out new ways of approaching problems and also reflecting back on how a particular attitude or way of behaving is likely to affect others.

People with cancer are often stunned when they realize what far-reaching effects the disease has – on partners, family relationships, beliefs and values. Even after treatment has apparently been successful and the family group is back together as before, there may be difficulties in communicating and problems with partners and children because of the anxiety and uncertainty caused by the cancer. Being natural no longer seems possible with everyone; as one woman described it, you are 'walking on egg-shells'.

Three years after an operation for bowel cancer one woman feels confident again and is leading a normal life. But her husband has remained permanently depressed, withdrawing from the family and refusing to make plans for the future. In another case a previously conscientious pupil has become disruptive and lazy since his mother went into hospital for a lumpectomy. He will not talk about his feelings to his parents and they do not know what to do.

These are the sort of situations in which counselling can help by uncovering the root of the problem – whether it is fear of loss, a feeling of helplessness or resentment at the disruption sickness causes. Those counselled often find that simply talking about a situation clarifies the possibilities and makes it easier to bear.

HOW DO I FIND A COUNSELLOR?

Your doctor may know of one, or even work with one; a minority of GPs now have counsellors in their practices. But you may prefer to go to someone quite independent, away from where you are known.

The British Association for Counselling (BAC) has more than 3000 individuals and 200 organizations in its membership and can supply names of people working in your area. Membership does not imply official recognition of an individual's competence but all members must assent to the Association's code of ethics. This states, among other things, that counsellors should inform clients about their training, qualifications and fees. BAC also have more than 200 accredited members, counsellors who have asked for their training and experience to be validated by a professional committee of the Association. In London, the Chelsea Pastoral Foundation provides specialist counselling for people with cancer and their families.

WILL I HAVE TO PAY?

Yes and no. Free counselling is not generally available on the NHS outside hospitals and it is normal for counsellors to charge something, but many vary their fees according to the client's ability to pay. Charges range from £10 up to £35 an hour. At the Chelsea Pastoral Foundation an individual session is normally £15, but, the Foundation stresses, nobody is excluded from counselling because of low income. Some clients pay 50p a session.

Unlike doctors, counsellors are not subject to a regulatory body like the General Medical Council, which lays down obligatory training, registration requirements and standards of professional conduct. In theory, at least, there is nothing to stop anyone setting up as a counsellor.

So the onus is on the client to find out what is being offered and on what basis. BAC suggests that new clients treat the first meeting with a counsellor as an opportunity to talk without obligation on either side. Feel free to ask anything you like and satisfy yourself that this is a person you feel able to trust, the Association advises. The first meeting should also include practical matters such as the length, place and cost of sessions.

USEFUL ADDRESSES

British Association of Cancer
United Patients
121–123 Charterhouse Street
London ECIM 6AA
Tel: 01-608 1661

Cancer Aid and Listening Line
The Gaddum Centre
274 Deansgate
Manchester
Tel: 061-434 9163/8668

Colostomy Welfare Group
38–39 Eccleston Square
(4th Floor)
London SWIV IPB
Tel: 01-828 5175

Breast Care and Mastectomy
Association
26 Harrison Street
London WCIH 8JG
Tel: 01-837 0908

CancerLink
46 Pentonville Road
London NI 9HF
Tel: 01-833 2451

Chelsea Pastoral Foundation
155A Kings Road
London SW3
Tel: 01-351 0839

British Association for
Counselling
37A Sheep Street
Rugby
Warwickshire CV21 3BX
Tel: 0788 78328

Cancer After Care and
Rehabilitation Society
Church Lane
Timsbury
Bath BA3 1LF
Tel: 0761 70731

Help for Health
South Block
Southampton General Hospital
Southampton SO9 4XY
Tel: 0703 777222 ext.3753
or 703 779091

Tenovus Cancer Information
Centre
11 Whitchurch Road
Cardiff CF4 3JN
Tel: 0222 619846

Bristol Cancer Help Centre
Grove House
Cornwallis Grove
Bristol BS8 4PG
Tel: 0272 743216

Cancercare Lancaster
Lancaster Royal Infirmary
Ashton Road
Lancaster LA1 4RP
Tel: 0524 381820

National Association of
Laryngectomee Clubs
4th Floor
39 Eccleston Square
London SW1V 1PB
Tel: 01-834 2857

Leukaemia Care Society
PO Box 82
Exeter
Devon EX2 5DP
Tel: 0392 218514

Women's National Cancer
Control Campaign
1 South Audley Street
London SW1Y 5DQ
Tel: 01-499 7532/4

Leukaemia Research Fund
43 Great Ormond Street
London WC1N 3JJ
Tel: 01-405 0101

Chapter Eight

JOINING A GROUP

WHAT HAPPENS AT A SUPPORT GROUP

'It can be quite inspiring just to hear how some people are coping. They're so determined not to be ground down, you think "well, I won't be either . . .".' (36-year-old cured of Hodgkin's disease)

'I don't know how I'll feel from day to day but it helps to come here. I like to see other people and hear how they're getting on . . .' (45-year-old woman with lung cancer)

'Whenever a patient mentioned joining any sort of group I thought how depressing, people sitting round discussing their problems all the time. But it isn't like that. It's very positive and we have some laughs.' (46-year-old GP who joined a group when recovering from breast cancer)

On a freezing February evening CancerLink Wimbledon is preparing for its regular meeting in a community hall. Members arriving in ones and twos arrange the chairs in a large circle. Every other meeting the group has a professional speaker – a doctor, nurse or social worker talking about some aspect of cancer. But this time it is the members' turn.

About twenty people turn up and the meeting starts with everyone saying a little about themselves. The group includes friends, partners and relatives and two radiographers from the Royal Marsden Hospital, as well as people who have, or have had, cancer.

An elderly man who has been coming to the group for several years says he does so to encourage others, as well as to meet people. Treated for lung cancer four years ago, he feels well and hopes others will find his recovery heartening.

Several people mention treatment undergone since the last meeting and how they reacted. One man who has had radiotherapy treatment explains that he is apprehensive about going into hospital for another scan, but feels more optimistic than a couple of months earlier. Members remark on how well he looks.

A woman with breast cancer and her husband tell the group they are worried about a sister-in-law who has never been in contact since she heard the diagnosis. Have other members had similar problems? And, if so, were they very hurt? Someone suggests they take the initiative and get in touch.

A young woman apologized for having missed the previous meeting because of babysitting problems. She comes because she is worried about her mother in the USA who has cancer and finds the group a good source of support. She is extremely concerned that her mother does not ask about the treatment she is having, and that her relatives are not doing enough.

Perhaps, suggests another member, 'forgetting' about the illness and living from day to day is her mother's way of coping. The young woman explains that she worries all the time and feels she should be with her mother. But with two young children that is more or less out of the question. Later one of the couples offers to look after the children whenever she decides to visit her mother.

The talk turns to coping with depression and 'down days'. Everyone in the group agrees that a good cry sometimes helps, 'just like a dose of salts'. But cosseting is also important, 'someone to listen who doesn't tell you to buck up'. Several people say how uplifting it can be to see people with cancer looking well.

A woman recovering from a hysterectomy and a course of radiotherapy explains that she still feels very much preoccupied by cancer, but that the group gives her a feeling of acceptance. Outside she worries about friends' and colleagues' reactions when she talks about her illness. But here she feels at ease about discussing treatments and side-effects because most people have been through similar experiences. The meetings give her a new perspective on her illness, she says. 'You see people with the same sort of problems as yourself, some of them very much worse and they are living with them and getting through their ups and downs . . .'

Others say that while the possibility of a recurrence is always at the back of their mind, it no longer preoccupies them all the time. One man says he never thinks of *having* cancer, but rather of cancer being an enemy, 'an enemy which isn't going to beat me'.

'I *had* cancer, it's in the past. I don't feel it's something hanging over me,' says a member who has undergone two operations. 'I feel well and I think that's very important.' Another woman suggests that keeping busy prevents brooding about previous setbacks.

One member, not present at this meeting, had suggested that there was too much talk about cancer and that some of the evenings should be purely social. The idea is rejected unanimously. Social evenings are easily come by elsewhere, the members feel. Their need is to share a special experience.

After a few false starts with the cassette player the meeting ends with a relaxation session. Everyone uncrosses their legs, shuts their eyes and tries to empty their minds of anxieties and distractions. The room falls silent but for the soothing voice of the leader, encouraging people to relax their bodies, part by part, until they feel a pleasant sense of warmth and heaviness. Afterwards members arrange lifts for those without transport.

WHY SUPPORT GROUPS HAVE BEEN SET UP

Given the prevalence of the disease it is strange that self-help for people with cancer is a comparatively recent development. There were groups for people with most medical conditions – alcoholics, gamblers and weight watchers – long before such things existed for the thousands living with cancer. It is really only in the last decade or so that cancer support groups have taken root.

One of the first of these was in Scotland. Realizing that the disease had implications far beyond what was seen on the wards and in out-patients' departments, Glasgow's Professor Ken Calman saw the need to bring together staff, patients and families. In 1980 he started a group at the city's Gartnavel General Hospital, known as Tak Tent (from the old Scots phrase for 'take care'). The network now incorporates more than a dozen community- and hospital-based groups, including two south of the border – at Homerton and St Bartholomew's Hospitals, London.

Professor Calman had noticed that patients wanted more opportunity to clarify details of their treatment, ask about cancer and talk about their feelings but felt guilty about taking up doctors' and nurses' time. And for their part the staff were frustrated that work pressures often prevented them from spending time with patients and families who obviously needed it. So he organized an evening meeting in a staff member's home, which was attended by some fifteen patients and relatives and a few hospital staff. Those who attended found the occasion helpful and it was decided to hold regular group meetings.

Another organisation, CancerLink, has established more than half-a-dozen groups of its own and also maintains a national directory of groups listing more than 100 organizations. Altogether more than 200 cancer self-help groups are believed to be underway in the UK, working in very different ways, with a variety of origins.

Very many have begun with an individual who felt a lack of support during or after cancer treatment and placed an advertisement in a local paper to test for others in the same predicament. Early meetings are often in the instigator's home, moving to community centres or permanent premises as interest grows. Most groups average about twenty people a meeting, although many are in touch with a circle of sixty or more.

As well as holding monthly or weekly meetings, some groups run telephone advice lines, staffed by trained volunteers, and operate home-visiting schemes, as well as visiting people when they are in hospital. Although some specialize in one type of patient, such as those who have had a mastectomy, the majority are open to people who have, or have had, any type of cancer.

Some groups, such as those in Tak Tent, are fairly structured, with formal management committees which include solicitors and accountants; others less so. Many change their ways of working according to who is in the group.

HOW TO FIND OUT ABOUT OTHER LOCAL GROUPS

If you feel you might like to join a group, or at least take a look, ask your GP or the doctor in charge of your hospital treatment what is available locally. In several areas consultants take the initiative and refer patients to groups. Some hospital departments, in contrast, will not allow a single leaflet or poster mentioning cancer to be displayed for fear of the effect on waiting patients.

If your doctor seems very negative when you suggest joining a group it is worth finding out why. Is it from ignorance or experience? There may be good reasons for avoiding a particular group, such as its 'pushing' one approach without regard to individual needs or previous treatment. Or the group may have become the vehicle for one person's preoccupations. But in some instances your doctor may simply have a hazy, uninformed view of what self-help in general, and cancer groups in particular, are all about. And that is no reason for you to be put off.

Dr Alison Edwards, a GP in Leicester, readily admits that before developing cancer herself she took a dim view of groups and was, as she puts it, 'wary of anything started in someone's back room'. But when she was recovering from a mastectomy she decided to investigate her local cancer support group and was struck by how positive and encouraging it felt. Far from the endless chewing over of difficulties that she suspected, she found acceptance, encouragement and humour. The warmth, friendship, caring and commitment of those involved have been a real inspiration, she says. Self-help, she stresses, needs to be seen at first hand to be fully appreciated. And doctors with no direct knowledge of groups are likely to persist in their belief that sharing experience creates problems rather than solves them.

So do not be put off simply because your doctor is unenthusiastic about groups. Look for other sources of information. Besides the British Association of Cancer United Patients (BACUP) and CancerLink, libraries, citizen's advice bureaux and community health councils are likely to have details of local groups. Where there is no cancer group underway they may have contacts interested in starting one. *Someone to Talk to*, a large self-help directory compiled by the Mental Health Foundation and published by Routledge and Kegan Paul (available in public libraries), lists more than 140 groups and organizations in its cancer section. Entries show the scope and services of each organization, and whether a membership fee is charged.

JOINING A GROUP – KEY QUESTIONS

Once you have made contact with a local group it is important to find out:

- Who goes? Just patients, or partners, families and friends?
- Where are the meetings? Can lifts be arranged for those with transport or mobility problems?
- Are there any doctors, nurses, or radiographers in the group?
- Does the group have access to specialist advice?
- Is any one approach promoted to members?
- Are members encouraged to continue with conventional cancer treatments?
- How does the group get its members? By referral? Word of mouth?
- Are there separate meetings for new members? Partners? Families?

After two or three meetings, deciding whether to remain will be a mixture of reason and gut reaction. It may help to ask yourself quite early on what you want from the meetings.

WHY DO PEOPLE JOIN SELF-HELP GROUPS?

Asked the question at the National Conference of Cancer Groups held at Keele University in April 1986 representatives listed (in this order): support, help, avoiding isolation, sharing experience, information, meeting others in the same position, opportunity to talk, a chance to be listened to, to plug the gap in health and social services, ego trips, social outlet, problem solving, feedback and care.

Most groups stress the importance of a holistic approach to cancer support, recognizing members' social, spiritual and emotional needs, as well as the practical and physical aspects of the disease. If, after a few meetings, you do not feel any better in any way – more encouraged, optimistic and less isolated – the group is probably not for you, however good the organizers' intentions. Most groups are at pains to point out that the support they offer is intended to be 'complementary' to established cancer treatments, not an alternative. None the less, many include people who have either abandoned, or decided against, the hospital treatment offered and their experiences will form part of the group discussions and may influence others who are deciding on how to handle their illness. There is nothing wrong with this. Groups exist to help people draw on the experiences of others who have 'been there'. And for every member who urges abandoning conventional cancer treatments there will be a dozen who oppose that view, urging people to accept as much help as possible. But groups who push one approach on all members, irrespective of what the individuals think, or feel, they need, are to be avoided. They have abandoned one of their main functions – to encourage people to make their own decisions.

WHAT A GROUP CAN DO FOR YOU

'I suppose you could talk to people in out-patients or while you are waiting for radiotherapy. But then you just want to get through with the treatment and go home. It's later you realize you need to meet people who have been through the same thing . . .' (36-year-old following treatment for Hodgkin's disease)

'I want to see people who are coping and getting on with life, several years on.' (Woman with breast cancer)

Even long after the treatment is completed many people feel the experience of cancer has changed their lives and outlook quite distinctly and that the disease has long-lasting effects on relationships. The possibility of a recurrence is always a concern, although anxiety about getting ill again diminishes with time.

Joining a group offers regular opportunities to talk about your experience of the disease and to benefit from the experience of others, including those who have been living with, or recovering from, cancer for several years.

Groups offer a 'sounding board' against which to test whatever you have been told about your disease and treatment. And, more importantly perhaps, they provide a sympathetic hearing and interest in members' progress which can be especially helpful for people living alone and for those who feel isolated. People in groups say that during down days it is encouraging to be able to look forward to the set monthly meeting when they will be able to share their feelings. And regular meetings can also help members chart their own progress.

For people recovering from the side-effects of treatment and who have lost confidence in their appearance joining a group can sometimes be a valuable stepping-stone back to normal social life, a safe setting in which to adjust to meeting new people.

Groups also offer a chance to be yourself and give vent to your feelings, whether that is very vocal anger, resentment or simple fatigue, without risk of offending anyone. This can be very helpful for those who are determinedly putting on a brave face for family and colleagues. Those who have had cancer know how deep and persistent are the feelings of loss and resentment and appreciate others' need to talk. Where groups are hospital-based they offer patients who think they may have to return at some point a chance to keep in touch with staff.

People with cancer often want their experience to benefit others and joining a group enables them to give active support. Members give as well as get, and groups can offset the feeling of passivity patients often have during, and immediately after, treatment.

Most groups are used to people coming alone because they 'do not want to worry' the family by talking about their disease. And more common still is the person who comes for advice about how to approach a partner who has clammed up and become completely uncommunicative since developing cancer.

Although women tend to predominate (as they do among callers to telephone advice services) groups normally include one or two couples who are happy to talk about the difficulties in partnerships and how they got around them. Their presence can be very reassuring to a partner who has come along to the group somewhat reluctantly. Some groups provide special meetings for partners and families and most are very much aware how easy it is for relatives' needs to get overlooked.

Cancer still has such strong and frightening connotations that families often feel all their anxieties and frustrations must be suppressed to ensure that maximum attention is given to the person with the disease. In reality this proves impossible and highly stressful. But families can experience huge guilt when they believe they have fallen short of what they should be doing, or feeling. Bewilderment, resentment, anger and sheer exhaustion are as common among partners and children as in those they are trying to support. And all too often there is no outlet for these emotions.

Groups offer a chance to air negative feelings that are never likely to be discussed within a charged family circle. And, at the very least, they provide evidence that others find these problems equally taxing. Bewildered by a sense of helplessness and fatigue, families and carers are reassured to see that others in the group feel this way too.

The experience of being part of a group can also encourage members to take a more active stance towards their illness, and towards their lives in general. Following the diagnosis of cancer it is very normal for people to become self-absorbed as they take in the implications of having a serious disease and gradually come to terms with it. But some people seem to get stuck, utterly pre-occupied by the knowledge that they have a potentially fatal disease. Groups can inspire people into a more positive frame of mind, encouraging members to take life a day at a time.

WILL IT BE DEPRESSING?

Depression is often noted by professional observers of the cancer self-help movement as one of the 'dangers' or drawbacks of groups. It can be very depressing when members weaken visibly or die, they warn. And, they suggest, a group that has endured a series of deaths is likely to remain subdued for some time. But those in groups feel that this is less of a problem than it might first appear from outside. They point out that part of the group's function is to help people come to terms with death and dying, and that the loss of a member through death does not always provoke depression and fear.

In some cases the group gets a feeling that someone is 'ready to go' and has chosen to accept rather than fight the disease. In such cases there is no sense of shock or failure. As one member put it: 'Death in a group isn't the awful numbing shock that outsiders seem to expect. You're sad, of course, but that doesn't stop the group functioning. People who absolutely can't tolerate the knowledge that cancer is linked to death probably wouldn't come to groups in the first place.'

But if, after several meetings, you go home more depressed than when you arrived, and voicing your feelings does not improve the situation, it is probably best to vote with your feet. At the risk of stating the obvious, groups exist for your benefit, not vice versa.

DO GROUPS WORK?

Some research on cancer self-help groups suggests they protect members from isolation and depression. A US study of 86 women with breast cancer showed those within a group had a greater feeling of control and suffered less depression and fatigue than those outside the group. And the rate at which groups are multiplying suggests that they fulfil a strong need. And those within them report that they feel their quality of life has improved, even if the benefits cannot be assessed objectively. Many people sense that a group may provide valuable support, even early on in treatment. At Homerton Hospital, London, anyone newly diagnosed with cancer gets a letter explaining that groups are available at the hospital and inviting them to a meeting. About one in five takes up the invitation.

Growing interest from health authorities is another indication that groups are beneficial for people coping with cancer. In some areas group members are allowed on to wards, to talk to patients who may later join.

At Walsgrave Hospital, Coventry, for instance, all women who have undergone a mastectomy are offered the chance to talk to someone from the local group who has had the same operation. In a five-year period more than 350 patients were helped in this way. And the Family Practitioner Committee, responsible for the family doctor service, distributes the group's leaflets to all GPs in the area, so they can tell patients what is available in the way of self-help.

Members of Merseyside Mastectomy Association have been invited to talk to student nurses. And the secretary of Tak Tent sits in the waiting room of the cancer clinic at Gartnavel Hospital to discuss the group's work and to answer queries that patients feel are too trivial for the doctor.

HOW PROFESSIONAL SHOULD GROUPS BE?

Within the cancer self-help movement there is lively disagreement about the best structures and orientation for groups and whether or not volunteers should be trained.

Many groups have a handful of members who have undergone some form of counselling course, but a significant proportion do not and resist a suggestion that training is necessary to help people in distress. You do not need a course in counselling to show that you care, is how one speaker at the National Conference at Keele University in 1986 put it. And many groups share her view that groups' amateur status is something to be cherished. Too much emphasis on formal training, it is feared, will produce 'them and us' divisions within groups, when the proper starting point should be sharing the common experience.

None the less, some groups insist on training for leaders, or 'key members' as they are called in Cancerlink groups. The Cancerlink training, which is open to people from other groups, consists of 12 three-hour sessions covering topics such as radiotherapy, nutrition and chemotherapy and communication skills. As well as importing basic knowledge about cancer and its treatments, training aims to make volunteers aware of their limitations and unafraid to admit their ignorance.

It is not volunteers' jobs to advise on treatments although they may clarify points of information. In its guidelines to groups Cancerlink points out that volunteers should not promote any one type of treatment to members, but rather support them in whatever treatment they are undergoing. And the guidelines also stress the importance of keeping a balanced view of the local cancer scene. Volunteers need to be able to see both the good points, as well as the deficiencies, in medical and other services, the guidance points out. Anyone thinking of joining a group should feel quite entitled to ask about its structure and whether or not any of those involved have been trained. Those in charge should be happy to explain the group's aims and principles.

The role of the professional in a self-help group also arouses strong feelings. Some groups maintain that health professionals in general, and doctors in particular, are too prone to keeping on their expert's hat when they join groups. Others feel that having a professional in the group gives other members a valuable 'in' to local services, as well as specialist knowledge, and that their presence can help close the 'them and us' feeling that still exists between groups and hospitals in some areas. Most groups seem willing to admit doctors, nurses, social workers and radiographers provided they come as people, not professionals, and resist any temptation to 'take over'.

Their presence can be beneficial to them. Radiographers and doctors who normally only see patients at their sickest and lowest find it very encouraging indeed to meet people when they are getting better and returning to ordinary life. This was illustrated at a meeting of a Tak Tent group in Scotland when a senior nurse explained how worried she often felt about giving patients treatments which, in the short term, made them feel ill and debilitated. Seldom seeing patients except when they were vomiting or nauseated she questioned the morality of making people 'ill' in order to help them. 'Now I see some of them here in between treatments, smiling, relating to others, coping. This helps me see the positive aspect of what I am doing, which before caused me so much guilt,' she said.

At their best, groups can play a very powerful role in closing the communication gap between people with cancer and the professionals looking after them.

HOW LONG SHOULD YOU STAY IN A GROUP?

Stay in a group as long as you feel it beneficial and enjoyable, which may be a question of weeks, months or years. Some long-standing members look on meetings simply as a night out, an opportunity to meet people with a common interest on a regular basis. And their open, sociable approach can be strong encouragement for new members who cannot believe that there will ever be a time when cancer does not overshadow every waking moment.

*

Leaving hospital after treatment for cancer of the tongue, Hilary Baker was keen to share her experience. She saw an advertisement in her local paper for people interested in starting a group, went along and became a founder member of Croydon Cancer Concern.

'I had a lot of support at home and they were very good at work but I did feel an indefinable urge to talk about my experience. Groups give you a chance to say "this is what happened and this is how I feel". That can be very relieving, especially if you arrive with a lot of grief and anger you've been holding in.

'I didn't join with the idea of helping other people but it gave me a lot of confidence when I found I could. Just listening can be very helpful, because in hospital there's often no time for that.

'And there's a feeling of companionship, whether or not you decide to talk about your illness. That is important when you are trying to regain your confidence.'

Hilary has been in the group for three years but envisages becoming less involved. 'As time goes on you assimilate the experience of having had cancer and feel less need to talk about it.' A health education officer, Hilary knew her way round the NHS pretty well before developing cancer, but being a patient gave her a different perspective. She feels groups can reduce the anxiety patients often feel when their treatment is finished and they are expected to return to 'normal' life.

Chapter Nine

SORTING OUT YOUR FINANCES

UNEXPECTED EXPENSES

Illness almost always involves unexpected expenses and some reduction in income; cancer is no exception. But help is available from a variety of sources and can sometimes be obtained at very short notice.

It is well worth visiting the hospital social worker as soon as possible after the diagnosis is made. Consulting a social worker does not imply that you are feckless, inadequate or poverty stricken, but may save you weeks of worry about where to go for practical and financial help. He or she will be able to assess your overall situation and advise on what benefits you and your family are eligible for, claim them on your behalf or assist you to claim. This is a very valuable short cut at a time of crisis. Careful budgeting is likely to be the last thing on your mind, but a social worker can advise on how to deal with debts which may arise. Some old hospitals are well endowed with special funds for easing hardship and the social worker will have access to these.

For general advice on what benefits you are entitled to contact your local citizens advice bureau (CAB; addresses in telephone directory). There are more than 900 CAB in the UK. The service is free.

SOURCES OF HELP

FARES

The cost of travelling to and from hospital every day for treatment can mount up to £50 a week and more. The sums are likely to be even larger for families making daily visits to someone in hospital.

Help is available from the Department of Health and Social Security (DHSS), the National Society for Cancer Relief (NSCR) and, where the patient is under 21, the Malcolm Sargent Cancer Fund for Children.

THE DHSS

The DHSS scheme, set out in leaflet H11 available from hospital receptions or your local DHSS office, provides help with fares and petrol costs to and from hospital for in-patients and out-patients. To qualify you must be on a low weekly income, that is, receiving supplementary benefit. You may also qualify if you are just above the supplementary benefit level.

Broadly speaking if you qualify under one of the above you are entitled to the cost of your fares on the cheapest form of transport. If no public transport is available you should receive the taxi fare to the nearest point at which you can get public transport. If your doctor says you need an escort their fares will also be met but a letter from the hospital will be required to support your case. If public transport *is* available but you choose to go by car, your petrol costs will only be covered up to the cost of the (second-class) fare. Where public transport is not available and you go by car, your full petrol costs can be covered.

VISITING PATIENTS IN HOSPITAL

The DHSS may meet or help towards the cost of visitors' fares as outlined above providing they are on supplementary benefit and are close relatives of the patient or a member of the household before hospitalization. Those who do not qualify for help with fares under the DHSS provisions should apply to the NSCR, or the hospital social worker may be aware of appropriate charitable trusts.

STATUTORY SICK PAY (SSP)

This is paid by employers to cover employees for up to 28 weeks of sickness. The amount you get is related to your average weekly earnings. SSP is normally paid at the same time and in the same way as wages. If you are unable to collect SSP as you would normally collect your wages, you can nominate someone else to do so, or ask to be sent a cheque. If you are still sick at the end of 28 weeks your employer should give you the DHSS transfer form SSP1(T) to help your switch to state help, normally invalidity benefit.

SICKNESS BENEFIT

If you are unemployed or self-employed and therefore do not qualify for SSP you may be entitled to sickness benefit for the first 28 weeks of incapacity. At the end of that time sickness benefit will be replaced by invalidity benefit if you are still unable to work. Sickness pay is usually dependent on your national insurance contributions in the last complete tax year before the start of the calendar year in which your claim begins. If you are receiving dialysis, radiotherapy or chemotherapy which stops you working for two or three days a week you should get sickness benefit for those days.

INVALIDITY BENEFIT

This replaces sickness benefit or SSP if you are still incapable of work after 28 weeks.

ATTENDANCE ALLOWANCE

This is a tax-free allowance for those who have needed a lot of looking after for at least six months. It is not means tested and you do not actually have to have someone looking after you to qualify. It is your need for attendance which decides your eligibility, not whether you get it. You can qualify even if you live alone. There are two rates of attendance allowance, with higher payments for those who need attendance both by day and by night.

Who qualifies?
You must be so severely incapacitated that for six months you have needed frequent help to walk and get about, eat or drink, go to the lavatory, wash, bath, dress and undress.

When to claim
It is advisable to put in a claim when you have needed such attention or supervision for three months, even though you won't actually get any money until the six months is up. The claim will take two or three months to be processed.

How to claim
Ask someone to get leaflet NI 205 from a DHSS office. Fill in the form and send it to your regional DHSS office (addresses on form). If you can't get hold of the form, don't delay or you risk losing benefit. Write to the DHSS and ask them to send you the leaflet, saying you wish to claim attendance allowance. Keep a copy of your letter. The date it was sent should be treated as the date of your claim.

After you have claimed, a doctor from the DHSS will visit you at home to assess your situation. This is standard practice and does not imply that your word is doubted.

Result of claim
You will be told the result of your claim in writing. If you are turned down on medical grounds, you have the right to ask for a review. And it may be well worth doing so. In 1984 more than half the people who asked for their cases to be reviewed, following a refusal, were successful in getting the attendance allowance. Your request for a review must be lodged, in writing and within three months of receiving the decision of your claim, with: Attendance Allowance Unit, DHSS, Norcross, Blackpool, Lancashire FY5 3TA.

If you have been turned down for attendance allowance on non-medical grounds you can appeal to the Social Security Appeal Tribunal within three months.

INVALID CARE ALLOWANCE (ICA)

This is paid to people of working age who cannot work because they have to stay at home to look after someone severely disabled. You do not have to be related to the disabled person to claim. The allowance is not means tested and no national insurance contributions are needed. ICA is taxable.

Besides the basic allowance, supplements are paid for a dependent wife or housekeeper and dependent children. You can receive ICA as well as attendance allowance and mobility allowance.

Who qualifies?

Age – men must be at least 16 and under 65. Women – at least 16 and under 60. Married women are entitled to claim ICA, and an unmarried woman living with a man as his wife can also claim.

You must be spending at least 35 hours a week caring for someone who receives attendance allowance, or constant allowance paid with a war or disablement pension or allowance under the Diseases Benefit Scheme. ICA is not payable if the person claiming does work which pays more than £12 a week (before tax).

How to claim

Fill in the form at the back of the ICA leaflet NI 212, available from DHSS offices. Send the form to: ICA Unit, DHSS, North Fylde Central Office, Norcross, Blackpool, Lancashire FY5 3TA.

ICA can be back-dated for up to three months, or up to 12 months if you can show good cause for a late claim. If you are refused the allowance, you can lodge an appeal with the ICA Unit within three months.

MOBILITY ALLOWANCE

Mobility allowance is for disabled people who are unable, or virtually unable, to walk and are likely to remain so for at least a year. It is not means tested and is tax free. No national insurance contributions are needed to qualify. People can get it whether or not they are working and whether or not they live at home. And they can spend it how they choose – towards buying or hiring a car, taxis or a wheel chair, for instance.

Who qualifies?

Those applying for the first time must be 5 or over and not yet 66. If you are 66 or older and have not claimed mobility allowance you cannot get it.

How to claim

Fill in leaflet NI 211 from the DHSS and send it to: DHSS, Mobility Allowance Unit, North Fylde Central Office, Norcross, Blackpool, Lancashire FY5 3TA. Claims cannot normally be backdated. In the majority of cases a medical examination is required and is arranged by the DHSS. Claimants who are turned down have the right of appeal.

You may also be eligible for the mobility allowance if the exertion of walking would risk a serious deterioration in your health, as in the case of people with serious lung or chest conditions.

FREE PRESCRIPTIONS

If you have a colostomy, ileostomy or laryngectomy you will not have to pay prescription charges on any drugs or dressings whether or not they are required for these conditions. Also exempt from prescription charges are: children under 16; pregnant women and women who have had a baby within the last 12 months; people receiving supplementary benefit, or family income supplement, and their dependants; women of 60 and over; and men of 65 and over. You could also qualify for free prescriptions if you are on a low income. Check your eligibility in the leaflet National Health Service Prescriptions (P11), available from DHSS offices, hospitals, doctors' surgeries, chemists and post offices.

SAVE WITH A SEASON TICKET

If you are going to need a lot of drugs or dressings but cannot get them free a 'season ticket' (prepayment certificate) may save you money. They are available for periods of four months and a year. Details are available on form FP95 from post offices, local DHSS offices, chemists or Family Practitioner Committees (Health Boards in Scotland).

FUNERALS

The simplest funeral costs over £500 and undertakers' fees can represent a considerable burden for the partner or family who is not prepared. If you think you may need financial help it is important to apply *before* arranging the funeral. It's almost impossible to reclaim the costs later.

Social security provides payments for 'reasonable' funeral costs for those on low incomes – usually enough to cover a simple coffin, a hearse, one car, undertakers', cemetery or crematorium fees, chaplain's and organist's charges and a 'reasonable' sum for flowers. Claims should normally be submitted with an estimate from the undertaker you have chosen. Where claims are accepted the DHSS will either send you a girocheque payable to the undertaker or pay the bill direct.

Where partners and families are unable to pay for a funeral and death has taken place in hospital the hospital can arrange for a free contract funeral. A local undertaker provides a basic service, often at a crematorium. In these cases it is usually up to the undertaker to decide the time and place of the funeral.

Help with funerals following death outside hospital

Local authorities have a duty to arrange the burial or cremation of any person who has died in their area (but not in hospital) where there are no relatives or friends able or willing to make the necessary arrangements. However, local authorities have no powers to reimburse burial costs where a third party has already arranged the funeral. Efforts will be made to find out whether there is any relative who could help pay for the funeral or whether the person who has died had the resources to pay.

The ways in which individual councils arrange matters vary greatly, but normally a council has an agreement with a local firm of undertakers for a simple funeral service which is usually a cremation. This usually consists of a simple coffin, no car, no flowers, no organ but with a minister of religion present.

HELP WITH MORTGAGE PAYMENTS

If you are claiming supplementary benefit you may be able to receive an allowance to help with the interest element of your mortgage. But this will be limited to 50 per cent of the interest repayments for the first sixteen weeks, except for the over-sixties. Your building society, social worker, or local DHSS office should know the latest position.

WILLS

Making a will is not an invitation to premature death but a basic consideration for those close to you. It will save those left behind countless difficulties and ensure that your assets are distributed as you intended.

Quite apart from the sums of money involved, failure to draw up a will is often interpreted by surviving partners and children as a lack of concern about their long-term well-being. So give some thought to what will happen after your death and make a will *now*.

Consult a solicitor. Trying to draw up a will on your own is false economy – the complications can be endless, and very expensive. Your affairs and your language are unlikely to be as straightforward as you imagine. The North American who completed his will in three words – 'all to mother' – left reams of complications as he always referred to his wife as mother. Both women wanted the money and it was the lawyers who profited. So see a solicitor to ensure that your wishes are recorded as clearly as possible. An objective eye will often pick up ambiguities you have not noticed. Inquire about charges before making an appointment with a solicitor, outlining your situation and asking for the likely fee in drawing up your will. Find out what the hourly charge is and how many hours' work your will is likely to involve.

Some sympathetic solicitors will draw up straightforward wills for pensioners for as little as £15, but the average fee is likely to be £30–£60 depending on how many hours, telephone calls and letters are involved.

Before going to the solicitor write down your full name and complete address and the full names and addresses of those you would like to benefit from your will (the beneficiaries). Consider whether you want the beneficiaries to benefit in a particular way. If they inherit *outright* on your death they can deal with that inheritance in any way they like. But you can limit the inheritance in some way, saying, for example, that the beneficiaries should be allowed the income from the capital for life, or until remarriage, or that they should only inherit at a specific age.

List specific objects: paintings, cutlery, silver, armchairs, rings, brooches, and the people you want them to go to. Draw up a list of your assets, including: post office savings accounts, premium bonds, stocks and shares, houses, life insurance policies and *where to find them* (with the bank, filed under 'insurance' in bottom drawer of filing cabinet, etc.).

Include a paragraph or two on whether you would like to be cremated or buried, and where. People often hope to save their relatives/beneficiaries the cost of a funeral by leaving their body to be used by students for anatomical examinations. But, in practice, people who have had cancer are rarely accepted for this purpose.

Bearing in mind that the cost of flowers at the average funeral is £500 you may prefer donations to be made to charities. If so, specify which, and be especially careful when it is a cancer charity. It is not enough to say 'cancer research' or 'for the benefit of people with cancer'; you need to name the charity and give the address if possible.

Where there are children under 18 it is extremely important to make guardianship arrangements and to record these in your will. Children should have two guardians – a natural parent, plus one other. You should also allow for the possibility that you and your partner might die together before the children have reached 18 by naming two guardians who would take over if that happened.

Executors

In your will you should name two people who have agreed to undertake the job of executors. They will be responsible, broadly speaking, for seeing that your wishes are carried out, as expressed in your will. This includes: arranging the funeral, paying debts and taxes, obtaining probate and seeing to the distribution of the estate. It is a good idea to appoint one professional executor – your solicitor or the bank's trustee department although a trustee department is likely to be more expensive than a solicitor – and one personal one – someone who knows where to find your belongings and will have time to sort out your clothes and kitchen cupboards.

The golden rule of making a will is be specific. Name the children, legitimate and illegitimate, whom you want to benefit and spell out your wife's/husband's full name. Take advice on ways of avoiding capital transfer tax at the time you make your will. It is a good idea to leave the will with the solicitor, with a copy at your bank and another at home.

MORTGAGES

If you are having difficulty meeting the monthly mortgage payments or foresee problems, contact the manager of the branch which arranged the mortgage and explain your situation. Building societies are sometimes prepared to suspend repayments for three months (especially when your case is explained in a report from a social worker) while you have a chance to sort out your financial position.

It may then be possible to extend the period of the mortgage so that there is less to pay each month. The building society may also agree to allow you to make interest-only payments, which will also lower the amount you have to pay. Extending the term of the loan is normally only possible with repayment mortgages. But it is possible to convert an endowment mortgage into a repayment one for an administrative charge of about £30.

Building societies stress that they will do everything possible to avoid repossessing your home for non-payment of the mortgage and would not generally apply to do so in under two years. But they want to know the reason for non-payment as soon as possible and the earlier you contact them the more sympathetic the response is likely to be.

Applying for a mortgage

Having had cancer should be no bar to obtaining a repayment mortgage, provided the building society is satisfied that your income is sufficient to meet the repayments. Where problems may arise is when you try to get some insurance – a mortgage protection policy – which will repay the amount borrowed in the event of your death. Insurers may either refuse your application altogether if the illness is very recent, accept it on condition that you pay a rated (higher) premium or suggest reapplying in six months or so. But people who have had cancer and appear to have been successfully treated are sometimes accepted for insurance without having to pay extra. And where a higher premium is required this may only be for a year or two.

Anyone who has had cancer and is applying for a mortgage protection policy or an insurance-linked mortgage will normally be asked to supply medical reports from the GP and consultant, and may also be asked to undergo a medical examination. The British Association of Cancer United Patients (BACUP) is in touch with brokers who have experience in placing mortgage applications from people who have had cancer.

INSURANCE

A diagnosis of cancer will not affect a policy already in operation prior to the illness. Finding a company to insure you once the disease has been diagnosed may be difficult, but it is worth shopping around. BACUP knows of sympathetic agents with experience in handling applications from people who have had cancer. Before considering your case companies will require medical evidence from your consultant. And if accepted you may be required to pay a loaded (higher) premium because of the extra risk you represent for the insurers. This higher rate may be charged as long as the policy remains in force, or the company may be willing to review the charge in accordance with your progress. After five 'clear' years the company may be willing to remove the loading and cover you at the normal rate. Companies unwilling to take you on during, or just after, treatment may look much more favourably at an application in a year's time. So keep looking.

The Association of British Insurers, a trade association representing more than 400 insurance companies, is happy to give general advice and guidance on insurance. They deal with over 2000 queries a year.

Travel insurance

Buying a fortnight's insurance at the same time as the holiday or air ticket is almost automatic and few of us go through the small print. But if you have, or have had, cancer you must say so and check what you are covered for in terms of medical expenses abroad, and transport home, should the need arise. Travel insurance generally covers medical expenses provided that the trip was not against doctors' advice and that the costs incurred are not for continuing treatment. Should you, for example, decide to break off your chemotherapy and go abroad for a week you would not be covered for chemotherapy while there. But in some cases companies may provide cover for such on-going treatment, provided that you give details of your condition when you apply for the insurance. Insurers will ask for a doctor's report.

Car insurance

There is no reason why people with cancer should be excluded. But you are required to inform the company of your diagnosis when the policy comes up for renewal.

HELP FROM CHARITIES

Cancer Relief

Cancer Relief (also known as the National Society for Cancer Relief) gives out more than £1.5 million a year in grants to people with cancer. Grants are made for: home-helps, sitters, home nursing, fares (for patient and family), nursing and convalescent homes, holidays, heating, clothing, bedding and special food, relatives' bed-and-breakfast costs, telephone installation and bills. The society provides cash for home comforts such as electric fires, fans, night tables, automatic kettles, electric blankets and liquidizers (for patients on special diets) and meets the costs of outings for people who would otherwise be housebound.

Applications normally go through social workers or community nurses but patients and families can apply direct. The Society arranges for the money to be given anonymously, so help can be given to those who do not know they have cancer. Grants are not normally given where the person concerned has more than £3000 in savings. But each case is considered on its merits and responses usually given within a few days.

The Society is very sensitive to the quality of life of people with cancer. A man preparing to welcome his wife back after hospital treatment was given a grant to redecorate their house. A former champion weight-lifter, confined to a wheel chair by his illness, was given help to buy a cordless telephone so that he could sit in his garden and still keep in touch. A young man who lost his job as a result of his illness and had to travel more than 20 miles for treatment was given money to tax his car. The Society does *not* make grants for the cost of private treatment.

Help can sometimes be given to terminally ill patients anxious to return to their country of origin and for relatives overseas to visit patients in this country. Where GPs see an urgent need for night or weekend home nursing the Society will sometimes agree to pay the costs before the formalities have been completed.

Malcolm Sargent Cancer Fund for Children
Since its establishment in 1968 the trust has helped more than 8000 families and finances social workers at more than twenty hospitals.

Help is available for anyone under 21 with cancer or leukaemia and grants are made for: travel costs, heating, toys, holidays, petrol, home nursing and bed and breakfast for parents visiting children in hospital. The Fund also makes subsistence allowances to single parents.

The fund is sympathetic to any request which will improve the quality of life for a child with cancer. An 18-year-old who underwent a bone marrow transplant for leukaemia was given help towards ballet lessons, as well as heating and travel expenses, to develop her interest in dance. There is no means test.

Application is normally through a hospital social worker.

The Joseph Rowntree Memorial Trust Family Fund

This fund provides help for children under 16 who are severely handicapped or dependent as a result of cancer, where similar support is not available from social services or social security. Grants are given for: washing machines (where the handicap produces a lot of extra washing), holidays for the whole family, outings, driving lessons (if a parent would then have regular access to a car), telephone installation and rental, clothing, bedding and recreational items.

Applications should be made direct to the fund.

Unions and professional societies

If you are a member of a union or professional society it is worth checking whether you are entitled to any benefits from that group and whether your family is eligible for any cash help. The Transport and General Workers' Union (TGWU), for instance, the largest union in the UK, with 1.4 million members, pays out invalidity benefit to members unable to work for up to ten weeks. And if you are a member of the TGWU and believe your cancer is related to your work the Union's legal department will investigate your case to establish whether you are entitled to compensation. The Union has won several compensation settlements of £20 000 where bladder cancer has been shown to have an industrial link.

Actors, bakers, bank employees, doctors, musicians, nurses, printers, social workers and teachers all have special benevolent funds which help with cash grants, and sometimes with holidays as well, in cases of hardship.

USEFUL ADDRESSES

The above and hundreds of other charitable sources are listed in the *Charities Digest*, published annually by the Family Welfare Association, 501–503 Kingsland Road, Dalston, London E8 4UA, and available in public libraries.

Cancer Relief
Anchor House
15/19 Britten Street
London SW3 3TZ
Tel: 01-351 7811

Joseph Rowntree Memorial
Trust Family Fund
PO Box 50
York YO1 1UY
Tel: 0904 21115

Association for British Insurers
Aldemary House
Queen Street
London EC4N 1TT
Tel: 01-248 4477

Malcolm Sargent Cancer Fund
for Children
14 Abingdon Road
London W8 6AF
Tel: 01-937 4548

Chapter Ten

KEEPING PAIN UNDER CONTROL

Just because you have cancer does not mean that you will suffer pain. One in three people with advanced cancer get no pain at all and for the vast majority of the others it can be kept totally under control. Better drugs and a greater understanding of pain and how to control it have meant that *no one* need suffer unbearable pain.

Yet many people with cancer fear pain more than anything else. Some admit that they are simply waiting for the pain to start. And relatives ask the doctors how soon they can expect it to begin. That is because we have all heard stories of how great uncle Percy had a tumour and died in agony. But we don't all hear of aunty Elsie who also has cancer and no pain at all; that's because she is getting on with life and does not have time to talk about the pain-killing drugs which she knows are there if she needs them.

Pain is no different from any other symptom. Like nausea, insomnia, diarrhoea or constipation it can be treated – and treated effectively. We all have our own ideas about what is painful. Some people are more sensitive to it than others. That does not make them weaker or less courageous, to be pitied or ignored. Pain is not something to feel ashamed about. Nor is it something to be judged against other people's ideas of what is painful. Pain is what *you* say hurts.

It is hardly surprising that someone with cancer dreads each unexpected twinge. A stiff neck – the result of lying awkwardly in bed one night – becomes a secondary tumour in the bones at the top of the spine; painful indigestion following a rather fatty meal becomes metastases in the liver. It is not just the fear of pain which haunts people with cancer; it is the knowledge of what the pain could mean – that the tumour has spread.

People do get pain from their primary tumour; it may be

what takes them to the doctor in the first place. But once their cancer has been treated, their symptoms, including pain, generally go away. Any sign that the pain has come back suggests that the cancer has also returned.

The only way to alleviate such fears is to find out exactly what is causing the pain. Once the stiff neck or indigestion is put into perspective it assumes the same lack of importance to someone with cancer as it would to anyone else. The pain itself frequently becomes less severe too. It is impossible to overstress the importance of putting your mind at rest. A few minutes' explanation about the cause of an unexpected ache or pain can save hours of anguish and fearing the worst. So don't keep your fears to yourself.

WHAT CAUSES PAIN IN CANCER?

Pain can occur for a variety of reasons. A tumour may block one of the tubes in the body. This can lead to a build-up of food in the gut, for example, or difficulty in passing urine if the tumour is obstructing the tube from the bladder. Either way, it will be painful until the tube is unblocked. People also feel pain when tumours press on other organs, especially if they trap nerves which are in the way.

Sometimes pain is felt some distance from the place where the tumour is pressing on a nerve. This is because nerve pathways join widely differing parts of the body. So pain caused by a tumour in the chest may be felt as pain in the shoulder or arm.

The difference between pain caused by primary tumours and pain arising from secondary tumours is not so much in the severity of the pain but in the way it is treated. Pain from primary tumours tends to disappear because the tumour is removed, whether by surgery, radiotherapy or drugs. Since secondary tumours are in general much harder to get rid of, the emphasis is on controlling the pain rather than on taking away the cause.

People with cancer also get muscle or joint pain, headaches or migraine just like the rest of us. But not only do they take on a new and often unfounded meaning — that the cancer has spread — they may aggravate other pains which really are due to the cancer.

Whether you get pain because of your cancer depends enormously on what type of tumour you have. But pain is not inevitable with even the most invasive cancers, and doctors marvel at patients who never have any pain despite large tumours pressing heavily on surrounding tissues.

Pain has a complex physical and psychological basis, and fear, tiredness, anger, depression and boredom are just a few of the feelings which can make it worse. Some people feel insulted if they think their doctor is looking for a psychological cause for their pain. There is nothing worse than someone not believing you when you are in pain.

'Do you think I'm a nutter, doctor?' is a common enough question. But it is not that the doctor doubts the pain; it is because pain is so complex that all the contributory factors must be found. Bucketsful of pain-killers will do little good in relieving the pain if anxiety or depression is at the root of the problem.

TELLING THE DOCTOR ABOUT YOUR PAIN

For you to get the most effective pain relief it is important to sketch as full a picture as possible about the particular pain you are suffering. Here is a brief guide to the type of questions you may be asked:

Where is the pain?
80 per cent of people with cancer pain complain of pain in more than one part of the body; some have as many as three or four distinct areas of pain. If it helps you to pin-point the areas draw a rough outline of the human body and shade the areas where you are getting pain.

Does anything relieve the pain or make it worse?
You may find that certain pains seem to occur at particular times of the day – in the evening, for example, when you are tired. Or they may worsen when you eat certain foods or when you move about. In contrast, sitting or standing in certain ways may alleviate the pain, or ice-packs or hot water bottles may help. You may already have tried simple pain-killers such as aspirin. Make a note or keep a diary of all the things which seem to affect your pain so that you remember them when you see the doctor.

What is the pain like?

Some pains are easy to describe, others less so. Try to remember whether you have ever had similar pains and what caused them. Is the pain a dull, continuous throb or does it come in sudden bursts which make you catch your breath?

Does it spread?

Pain sometimes starts in one part of the body and slowly spreads out – it may go down an arm or leg, or seem to give a burning sensation across your chest or abdomen. Once it has spread, does it stay there? Or do you wake up the next morning with the original pain, which then spreads during the course of the day?

How severe is the pain?

Give the pain a rating on a score of one to ten. Things to take into consideration would be: is it short and stabbing or dull and aching? Does it stop you in your tracks or prevent you from getting about and doing what you want to do? Does it affect your appetite or keep you awake at night? How does it compare with other pains you have had in the past, before or since your cancer was diagnosed?

Is the pain there all the time?

Does it come and go? Again, try and make a note of when you are in pain and when you are feeling better. Make sure that the doctor or nurse knows if you suddenly develop a new pain. It may need different treatment from that which you are receiving for pain in other parts of your body. Each new pain needs to be assessed along the lines outlined above so that you can get the most effective treatment.

HOW TO GET EFFECTIVE PAIN RELIEF

It is thought that around a quarter of people with advanced cancer do not get sufficient pain relief; both doctors and patients are responsible. On the patient's side there is the mistaken belief that pain is inevitable; then there are people who are so determined to be brave that they suffer in silence. Some do not like taking drugs or are worried that side-effects will make them dozy and unable to concentrate. Others fear that if they take them too soon the drugs will lose their effectiveness later on if the pain gets worse; this is a very common misconception.

Perhaps surprisingly, some doctors and nurses have similar, misguided fears. They too may be worried about prescribing painkilling drugs because the doses may be higher than they would normally use for other illnesses. They may be worried about side-effects and addiction to the more powerful drugs because they simply don't know enough about the use of pain-killing drugs in cancer. This can happen both in hospital and at home, in the care of the G P.

Like any other area of medicine, the treatment of cancer pain requires specialist knowledge and experience. An average G P is likely to see eight or ten cases of cancer a year and only a handful needing treatment for cancer pain. It is therefore hardly surprising that the G P is less attuned to dealing with people with cancer pain than specialists managing the problem every working day. Nevertheless, a lot of progress has been made in the last few years in getting the message across – that no one with cancer needs to be in unbearable pain. The vast majority need suffer no pain at all, and a tiny proportion may have to live with some discomfort, but not unbearable pain.

Who will advise you on pain control depends on where and when your pain starts. If you are in hospital then the doctors there will prescribe the necessary pain-killers or other treatment. If you are at home it will be up to your G P. The onus will be on you to tell whoever is caring for you how bad your pain is and whether the treatment is working. Non-specialists are getting better at controlling cancer pain, but if you are in difficulty you can ask for specialist help.

A growing number of hospitals around the country have either continuing care units or pain clinics attached to them. Initially you will be referred to a pain specialist to sort out your immediate problems. If you are in severe pain then your G P should be able to get someone to see you straightaway. If it is more of an intermittent problem then you will get an appointment depending on the length of waiting lists.

What happens next will depend on the service offered by your hospital. Some pain clinics have a home service with nurses who will come out and see you, or they have emergency telephone numbers if you run into problems. Those which work on a nine to five basis will leave you to call your G P if you are having problems. If you are referred to one of these hospital units the important thing is to find out exactly what the system is for emergencies. Be sure you know whether you should be ringing your G P or the unit. Don't wait until you need help in the middle of the night to find out!

If there is no hospital-based clinic in your area there may be either a hospice or a continuing care unit staffed by Macmillan nurses. These services are described more fully in the next chapter. But be aware that you do not have to be an in-patient to get help for pain problems from hospices or Macmillan units. Many of them have home-care teams. They may recommend that you go into the unit for a few days to get the pain sorted out and when you go home they will come to see that you are coping all right. You will be given an emergency telephone number to get help any time of the day or night.

The hospice and Macmillan teams specialize in all aspects of continuing care, not just pain relief. So you can discuss anything physical or emotional with them. For both these services you will need a referral letter from your G P. If you do opt for Macmillan care your G P will not wash his hands of you, but you should take all your pain problems to the Macmillan service as they will know what drugs you are taking and how you are getting on.

Many G Ps work closely with their local Macmillan or hospice service so will be kept in touch with how you are getting on. But they will not be as up to date with your progress as the nurses who see you on a daily or twice-weekly basis.

If your G P does not know what pain control services are available in your area you can contact one of the support services, described in the next chapter, which may have information about getting help in your area.

WHAT PAIN CONTROL MEANS

Treatment of cancer pain does not mean mind-blowing doses of 'hard drugs'! It means the relief of all the factors, physical and psychological, which contribute to pain.

Fear of the unknown is the biggest enemy. An understanding of what is causing the pain – even if this is the cancer itself – at least puts you on the right path to relief. The fact that someone is taking the pain seriously is important; even the knowledge that the pain has been investigated can take away some of the fear which may have been aggravating the pain.

Tea and sympathy won't make the pain evaporate, but when you are in pain there is nothing worse than feeling that no one is taking it seriously or that someone is doubting its severity. Just because someone in the next bed with the same type of cancer is free of pain does not make your pain any less real. It cannot be said too often that pain is what *you* say hurts.

A number of simple measures can be taken alone or alongside drugs to reduce both physical and psychological components of pain.. These are described next.

EASING PHYSICAL PAIN

Comfort

Check that some of the pain is not due to the way you are sitting or lying. Supports, in the form of pillows and specially shaped foam for the neck, can do wonders for many aches and pains. Foot stools can take the pressure off sore feet. If the bedclothes feel heavy try a lightweight duvet or ask for a frame to be put over your legs to keep the bedclothes raised. Many people who spend long periods sitting or lying down find that their bottoms get sore, particularly if they have lost weight, because the skin is constantly rubbing against clothing or bedding. Sitting on a rubber ring or lying on a sheepskin (both available through the National Health Service) can relieve this problem and prevent the development of open pressure sores.

It is very important to try and avoid sores. They occur when the top layers of the skin are rubbed away and the layers underneath start to break down. The sores can become quite deep, bringing the risk of infection, and they are very difficult to heal. They are most common in places where the skin is normally thinnest and is most likely to rub against clothing or bedding. This means elbows, knees, ankles and especially the base of the spine. Not spending too long with any one area of skin in contact with the bed or chair is the best way of preventing pressure sores, and also helpful is moisturizing cream rubbed regularly into areas which are at risk, especially if there are any signs of redness.

Hot water bottles, ice-packs and cushions placed on painful parts can bring instant and highly effective relief, particularly from joint, muscle and nerve pains. We have all used hot water bottles for backache and ice-packs to reduce swelling; even the pressure of a hand or cushion against the face can help relieve toothache. But these simple remedies are often forgotten when it comes to someone with cancer.

Relaxation

Like ice-packs and hot water bottles, relaxation techniques will not block out severe physical pain, but they can help to remove the stress component to pain and so act as a booster to drug and other methods of pain control. Relaxation exercises take many forms and every teacher has his or her own method. But three basic techniques are in general use: progressive relaxation, autogenic training and imaging. Progressive relaxation involves getting to know particular groups of muscles around the body. Once you become aware that you can relax and contract stomach muscles, neck muscles and all the rest individually or together you can start using the technique during stressful periods to reduce tension. Autogenic training encourages relaxation 'from within'. Relaxation of each part of the body – arms, legs, hands, feet, fingers, toes – is accompanied by thoughts of space, heaviness or warmth within those areas. The idea is that once the techniques are mastered you can go onto 'automatic pilot' from time to time so that your mind and body are functioning but you are relaxed and unstressed. Imaging relies on you being able to conjure up happy, relaxed pictures in your mind – deserted golden beaches, the sea lapping at your feet, tranquil valleys, the sounds of nature, the sun's warmth on your back.

Nerve stimulation

This has been used for thousands of years to relieve pain of all types, but there are doubts over its value in treating cancer pain. It is probably most useful where there are particular trigger points for the pain – when touching a particular point always causes pain either in that area or further away. Even so, most pain specialists would prefer to inject anaesthetic into such trigger points rather than use nerve stimulation. However, if you want to give acupuncture a try or have found it helpful with other conditions in the past, there is nothing to stop you. Try to get a recommendation or contact the Institute for Complementary Medicine (address at end of chapter) for the name of a reputable acupuncturist. Expect to pay £10–15 per session.

Nerve blocks

There are a variety of ways of stopping nerves from transmitting pain and these are especially useful in such things as facial neuralgia or the pain arising from cancers of the head and neck. Nerves can be blocked by injections of anaesthetic or by actually destroying them with chemicals or with heat or cold. All of these techniques have their place; the nerves do grow back, slowly, but nerve blocks can be very useful both in treating the specific types of pain mentioned above and for people who do not seem to respond to pain-killing drugs.

Radiotherapy

People whose pain is caused by secondary tumours in bones can get a lot of relief from a single dose of radiotherapy. Breast, lung and prostate cancers can spread to the spine, femur, pelvis and breastbone. The metastases slowly erode the bone and not only cause pain but also make the bones very brittle and easily broken. In destroying part or all of the secondary tumour, radiotherapy not only helps to relieve the pain, it also enables the bone to recalcify and return to its normal strength. It may not be possible to get rid of all of the cancer but radiotherapy can get rid of the pain and make you feel better.

EASING EMOTIONAL PAIN

Fear, anger, sorrow – all perfectly natural emotions for someone with cancer, but each with the potential to aggravate pain: worry about finances and how the family is coping; anger at bureaucratic delays in getting help from the social services; depression over the sense of helplessness; and, to make everything worse, endless hours of sleeplessness spent thinking about all those problems through the night. Friends and relatives can play a big part in finding and sorting out many of the worries faced by someone with cancer. They have the physical strength to badger authorities into unravelling bureaucratic red tape and they have the emotional reserves to reassure and dispel unnecessary personal worries.

The first hurdle is for you, the friend or relative, to get to the root of the anxieties.

The illness itself

Try to find out if there are any particular aspects of the illness which are upsetting to the cancer patient. They may be wondering whether there will be further treatment – surgery, radiotherapy or chemotherapy – and perhaps worrying about side-effects. Or they may feel that they have been 'written off' if no further treatment is proposed. They may not have been told the results of routine tests and be reading something sinister into this.

Who will be looking after the patient?

Many people with advanced cancers alternate between periods in hospital, hospice and home. After a few weeks of the routine of hospital they become nervous about going home and about whether they and their family will be able to cope. By going through the preparations which are being made at home, and the medical and social support which are available, many of these fears can be dispelled. Likewise, someone going into hospital may be worried that 'this is it'. A few words of explanation about what is being done and encouragement about going home when there is some improvement can take away the fear of hospital or hospice.

Financial implications

Some people with advanced cancer may want to go through the financial provisions for their family, both while they are ill and in case they die. It is easy to dissuade them from discussing such details, but this may take away their peace of mind that all is well. Equally, if the family's financial situation is less secure it may be just as important to find out what benefits will be available for the family so that the sick relative can be reassured that his family will not be left without a roof over their heads.

Spiritual unrest

Even the least religious people often look for spiritual help when they feel that they are dying. Hospital chaplains are very good at finding out if people do want help, but relatives may also be able to pick up on such needs and alert the relevant people.

Feelings of uselessness

Anyone who has been used to a central role in the events of a family is bound to feel unwanted when he or she can no longer fulfil that role. It is important to involve the relative with cancer in family discussions and decisions wherever possible and to keep them informed of family events: a favourite niece getting married, a neighbour moving house, redecorating the living room; all everyday events which are easily overlooked or not thought worthy of mention. But to someone who is very ill such oversight can easily signal 'out of sight, out of mind'.

GETTING THE DRUGS RIGHT

Choosing a pain-killer depends very much on the type of pain being treated. Either you can treat the pain where it is being caused – in the bone, muscle or nerve – or you can block the point at which the pain is registered – in the brain.

The humble aspirin is the first option for mild pain, whatever the cause. A form which dissolves in water is best because it is least likely to irritate the stomach. Aspirin should not be taken on an empty stomach for the same reason. Doses of up to 600 mg every four hours (the same as you would take for a headache or rheumatic pain) are recommended. Aspirin works by blocking the release of chemicals at the site of the pain.

Paracetamol is a useful alternative for anyone who suffers from stomach problems. Elderly people in particular have been shown to be at risk of ulcers and stomach bleeding if they take aspirin-like drugs, and so paracetamol is frequently a useful alternative – again preferably taken in soluble form in doses up to one gram (two tablets of most standard preparations) every six hours.

Aspirin, or one of the family of drugs which works in a similar way, is also the best option when the pain is definitely caused by inflammation of muscles or joints. This can occur as an indirect result of the cancer or it may be an entirely separate but coincidental pain. How you describe your pain will help the doctor judge what is happening. Not only does aspirin relieve the pain, it also reduces the swelling and inflammation – something which paracetamol cannot do on its own. There are many aspirin-like products in this group and you could just as easily be prescribed naproxen, ibuprofen or one of the others. As people vary in their responses to these drugs the doctor may try out several of them to see which works best.

WHAT HAPPENS IF THE PAIN GETS WORSE?

If the aspirin-like drugs do not ease your pain you are likely to be prescribed one of the drugs which acts centrally in the brain to block pain, instead of locally where it is being caused. Codeine or Distalgesic are most commonly prescribed. They are not just for cancer pain and are used routinely for a large number of painful conditions from back pain to post-operative pain. Both drugs are likely to be prescribed in higher doses than for other types of pain; they may make you feel drowsy, so you should be careful about driving or using potentially dangerous equipment such as lawnmowers, saws or electric carving knives.

Many people with cancer find that one of these drugs keeps them pain-free for many months and they need no further medication. Others find the drugs helpful for some time and then begin to find the pain breaking through. Continuing up this staircase of increasingly powerful pain-killing drugs, the next step is generally morphine, or its close relation, diamorphine. Tablet and liquid forms of morphine are now used more commonly than injections, which tend only to be given if there is a problem with swallowing. The reason it used to be given by injection was that it was thought to be poorly absorbed in the stomach and needed direct entry into the bloodstream. This has proved wrong for the vast majority of people, and for those few with absorption problems there is the additional option of morphine suppositories.

WON'T I GET ADDICTED?

There is simply no comparison between the way that morphine is used to relieve pain and the way that heroin is used to get high. For a start, the doses of morphine used in pain control are generally far lower than those used by addicts. The drug is likely to be purer and less likely to cause side-effects than the impure mixture used by addicts. And it is given by mouth rather than directly into the bloodstream.

Morphine rarely causes the kind of euphoria in people with cancer pain that it does in drug addicts. This is because in cancer pain the morphine is being used to correct an imbalance and to bring the sufferer back up to the normal, pain-free state. In the drug addict, who is in no pain, the effect is to overcompensate and raise the mental awareness of emotional state to hyperactive level. It is really no different from giving supplements to someone with an underactive thyroid to enable them to function at a normal rate. If you gave those same supplements to someone with a normal thyroid they would start to show all the hyperactive behaviour of someone with an overactive thyroid.

So people with cancer pain who are given morphine do not become mentally addicted to the drug, though they may become 'physically dependent'. This means that they could suffer physical symptoms and feel very unwell if the drug is stopped suddenly. Like so many drugs, the dose of morphine has to be reduced slowly to prevent withdrawal effects. This is no different from the precautions taken in reducing the dose of drugs for lowering blood pressure, the dose of steroids for arthritis or the dose of sleeping pills for insomnia. It is routine.

Again, like most drugs, it is normal to start with relatively low doses of morphine and to gradually build up. This does not mean that the doses will need to be increased indefinitely as the patient becomes tolerant to each new dose. Most people need the dose to be increased in the first days or week until their ideal dose is found. They then stay at that dose for perhaps weeks or months. If, then, their cancer is more advanced they may need more drug for effective pain relief. People vary enormously in their responses to morphine. One person may need only a fraction of the amount needed by the person in the next bed. Both can be equally free of pain on their medication, equally active and equally coherent and responsive.

YOU SHOULD NOT HAVE TO ASK FOR THE NEXT DOSE

Not only is it important to find the ideal dose of morphine, it is vital to get the timing right. No one should have to watch the clock between doses, terrified that their pain will return before the next dose is due. If the pain relief runs out between doses then the doses are not high enough and need some adjusting. Doses should be at regular intervals – not 'as required'. No one should be left to tell the medical staff when they are in pain; that will lead to inevitable delays in relief.

The key to effective pain relief in all chronic illnesses is: 'Don't wait until the pain comes back, catch it before the last dose of pain-killer wears off.' Remember, you don't have to prove that the pain is still there. So insist, or if you don't feel up to it get a friend or relative to insist, that the doctors and nurses get the doses and timing of your drugs right.

If you are at home it should be just as easy to tailor your drugs to your needs. There may be a few problems at the start, but once the doses and timing are worked out to suit you, your pain should be as well controlled as if you were in hospital or hospice. Be sure you know how to get help at any time of the day or night in case your pain does get worse and you need the doses changed.

Although four-hourly doses of morphine are the mainstay of relief of severe cancer pain, some people benefit from tablets which slowly release their contents over twelve hours. Another alternative is to fit a pump which slowly drips morphine under the skin. This is only really necessary for people who do not respond well to morphine given by mouth. A needle is inserted under the skin, often on the chest. This is linked to a syringe of morphine which is attached to a clockwork pump strapped to the shoulder or fixed into a pocket. The morphine is injected slowly and continuously at a pre-set rate. The syringe is refilled every day, or less often with some newer systems. The rate at which the morphine drips through can be speeded up or slowed down according to the severity of the pain.

You only have to talk to a few people taking morphine for cancer pain to realize that they do not sink into a hazy world of their own the moment the first dose of morphine is given. Reactions do vary and a handful of people find themselves feeling sleepy, particularly when the drug is first started, but many people are at home carrying on a relatively full and active life on quite high doses of morphine. Their thinking is clear and because they are not in pain they find that they can do far more than when their pain was not controlled by the morphine.

TREATING THE SIDE-EFFECTS OF MORPHINE

Morphine has two side-effects which will probably need treatment. The drug can make you feel sick, particularly in the first days of treatment, so an anti-sickness drug is generally prescribed until the nausea disappears. Morphine also causes constipation and so it is important to take a laxative to ensure that the bowels move every day. Constipation itself can be a very painful condition and in severe cases carries a risk of bowel obstruction, so laxatives are a routine part of morphine treatment.

Morphine is of course a highly effective pain-killer, but it may still be necessary to continue with other drugs working locally against pain. Some people find it rather strange that they are pre-scribed morphine and soluble aspirin – after all, as far as they are concerned, morphine is the most powerful pain-killer we have and wonder what something as simple as aspirin can do which morphine can't.

The answer is that, while morphine is extremely good at

blocking pain centrally in the brain, it is far less good at controlling pain and inflammation in joints and muscles. Aspirin, while having no effect on the brain, is very good in muscles and joints. So the two drugs complement each other and attack different types of pain and they are frequently given together.

OTHER DRUGS YOU MAY BE PRESCRIBED

You may also be prescribed tranquillizers and sleeping pills; as already mentioned, anxiety and insomnia can aggravate cancer pain. With the best will in the world, most people will be left with some worries about what is going to happen to them. So it seems quite sensible to take small amounts of tranquillizers such as diazepam (Valium) during the day and sleeping pills such as temazepam at night. Of course, if you are not anxious and you are sleeping all right there is no need for such drugs, but for some people they are very helpful.

Depression can also lower the amount of pain you can put up with and make everything seem worse. Talking over what is making you depressed can help, but if the depression is playing a major part in the pain you are getting from the cancer it is much more sensible to take anti-depressant drugs than to increase the dose of pain-killers, which may still not be effective.

You may well be taking a variety of other drugs for conditions unrelated to the cancer. High blood pressure and diabetes, for example, do not go away because you have cancer, and your regular treatment will continue. This can mean that you finish up taking a number of different tablets during the course of the day – perhaps as many as six or seven different drugs. In hospital, these are brought round regularly, but back home it will be up to you or your friends or relatives to make sure that you take them all on time. So how can you ensure that you get it right?

COPING WITH DRUGS AT HOME

Be reassured that you will not simply be discharged from hospital with your bottles of drugs and left to get on with it. Either you will return to the care of your GP and your local district nurses or you may be referred to the home-care team of your local Macmillan nursing scheme. If it does look as though the medical services have not been alerted to your return home shout loudly in the direction of your GP, or better still check what has been arranged for you before you leave hospital. You should certainly not leave hospital without you or a person caring for you knowing exactly what medicines have been prescribed for you and when and how to take them.

To ensure that you do take all your drugs regularly the first thing to do is to make a chart of all the medicines and when they should be taken. (Ideally, this should be done by whoever has given you the drugs to take home.)

It is important to streamline your tablet-taking or else you may find you are taking different sorts of tablets every one or two hours. So wherever possible it is advisable to time the doses so that you take several different drugs at the same time of day. If one of the medicines has to be taken only once or twice during the day then try to coincide it with one of the other drugs which has to be taken more often. By taking more than one medicine at a time you can cut down on the number of times per day you have to remember to take your medicines.

Put the medicines somewhere easily visible so that the sight of them will help to jog your memory and, if you are worried about remembering to take them, leave room on your chart to tick off each dose as you take it. As you probably won't want to make a new chart each day put a line through your row of ticks at the end of each day, or first thing the next morning, so that you know where you are.

If you find that you cannot cope – and lots of people can't, so don't feel embarrassed – talk it over with your GP, district nurse or health visitor and work out some system of remembering. Perhaps friends and relatives can pop in to make sure that you are taking the medicines regularly, or nurses can visit two or three times a day to see that all is well. It may all seem rather confusing to start with but, like anything else, it will seem much easier once you get the hang of it.

The golden rule is that whether you are in hospital, in a hospice or at home you should not be in pain.

USEFUL ADDRESS

Institute for Complementary Medicine
21 Portland Place
London WIN 3AF
Tel: 01-636 9543

Chapter Eleven

HOME, HOSPITAL, HOSPICE?

'A dying person is a living person.' (hospice philosophy)

'It is impossible to overestimate how precious life is to the dying.'
(Macmillan nurse)

Progress in pain relief and the rapid growth of the hospice movement in the last twenty years are among this century's most humanitarian advances. Care of the dying now attracts considerable medical debate and enormous charitable enthusiasm, with almost every community looking for ways to start its own hospice or home-care team.

This is not without its problems and there is concern about the long-term security of hospices if the National Health Service (NHS) cannot be persuaded to pick up a larger share of the bill. Health authorities meet less than half the running costs of the 100 or so hospices operating in the UK, and even the most ardent champions of hospice care see the need for a national, co-ordinating plan. It is unreasonable, they say, for local fund-raisers to build their hospice without consultation and then expect the health authorities to pay for the running costs.

But from the point of view of the person with advanced cancer the proliferation of hospices and their ideals has brought nothing but good. The aims of the hospice movement – involving the family in the caring as well as catering to the physical, emotional and spiritual needs of the patient – have spread beyond the units themselves to be taken up by general hospitals and staff looking after the dying at home.

Hospice care is now provided by specialist units in general hospitals and by about 100 home-care teams, as well as in hospices themselves. Most deaths from cancer take place in hospital, but about a third are at home and 10 per cent in hospices. But this does not mean that most people with cancer spend all their last weeks in hospital. Many are cared for at home almost up to death and many have a combination of hospital, hospice and home care. Where someone is cared for depends on personal and family choice, geography, home circumstances, doctors' preferences and the progress of the disease.

There is general agreement about what makes for a peaceful end and a good death: dignity, family support, freedom from pain, control of distressing symptoms, security and the time to make peace with the world. But the best place for that will vary according to the person. Some people are adamant that they want to stay in familiar surroundings come what may and pursue that aim determinedly and successfully even when living alone with virtually no support. For these people remaining at home overrides the possible advantages of constant medical supervision and the assured regularity of life as an in-patient.

Others decide on hospital or hospice admission, after weeks or months of being looked after at home, because they are insecure about their pain being controlled, or are worried about the strain on the person looking after them. Some people are content or resigned to staying or returning to the hospital where they have received most of their treatment. But others are anxious to get away from a place which may have unpleasant associations of debilitating treatment. And for these people home care may be the answer. This chapter outlines hospice and home care.

WHAT IS A HOSPICE?

Originally a place of rest and sustenance for medieval pilgrims, the term now refers to a small, specialized unit caring for the dying and those with incurable illness.

There are more than 100 such units in the UK, ranging from the sixty-bed St Christopher's Hospice in Sydenham, South London, which pioneered many of the ideas now prevalent in palliative cancer care, to Helen House, the eight-bed children's hospice in Oxford. St Joseph's, Hackney, the first hospice in the UK, founded by the Irish Sisters of Charity in 1905, has more than 100 beds. But the newer ones, most of which have been built in the last twenty years, are very much smaller. The average size is 20–30 beds. Most hospices were built by charities, but the NHS now helps towards the running costs in many cases.

The term hospice also includes:

- Macmillan continuing care homes – units built in the grounds of the NHS hospitals, with the charity, Cancer Relief, providing the capital and the NHS paying the running costs.
- Sue Ryder Homes which look after severely disabled people as well as those with advanced cancer.
- Marie Curie residential nursing homes for people with cancer.
- Continuing care wards in NHS hospitals – specialist units devoted to the care of the incurably ill.

Hospices aim for a calm, peaceful atmosphere involving the relatives in the care of the sick person. The staff/patient ratio is often higher than in hospitals and the emphasis is on quality of life. Considerably more informal than hospitals, most hospices have no restrictions on visiting times. The accommodation is usually a mixture of small wards and single rooms. Many run some sort of bereavement programme, including group meetings or visits to the partner or family after a death.

HOME-CARE TEAMS

In addition to these residential hospices there are about 100 home-care teams operating in the UK. These bring hospice-type nursing to people being looked after in their own surroundings. About half these teams are attached to hospices or hospitals while the remainder are based in the community. Most have access to beds in a hospice or in a community or general hospital when they have someone who needs in-patient care.

Home-care teams normally consist of two to six specially trained nurses and they generally work alongside, or in liaison with, GPs and district nurses. The home-care team at Trinity Hospice, South London, for example, sees some 200 new patients a year, with referrals coming from GPs, hospital consultants, district nurses and social workers. Three nurses and a doctor look after some forty families at any one time, with every patient visited or contacted by telephone at least once a week, and medical staff taking turns for evening and night calls. The nurses are in contact with district nurses and GPs who give the patients day-to-day care and can arrange admission to a hospice when necessary.

In addition, several general hospitals, such as St Thomas's in London have teams which offer specialist advice on pain control and palliative care to doctors within the hospital and to GPs looking after people who have cancer and are living at home.

DO PEOPLE ONLY GO INTO HOSPICES TO DIE?

No. It is quite normal for people to go into hospices for short periods during which time their symptoms are monitored and brought under control; then they return home. A short stay in a hospice, where specialist care and advice is available, is often the quickest way of relieving pain and problems such as diarrhoea and vomiting. Response to drugs can be followed closely by staff giving continuous care in a way that is not possible while the person is at home.

Hospices also admit people in order to give relatives and carers a break for a weekend or longer. A short-term admission to the hospice enables the family to rest and catch up on sleep, secure in the knowledge that their relative is being well looked after.

Will there be a waiting list?

No, not in the hospital sense. Pressure on hospice beds is nothing like that on hospital beds and it is very unlikely you would have to wait more than a week or two for admission. Many hospices have emergency beds for people who need admission at very short notice, because they have deteriorated suddenly or relatives are very strained.

Will I have to pay?

No. Free care for those in need is one of the fundamental principles of the hospice movement. But donations are always welcome.

How can I find out if there is a hospice nearby?

Through your GP, hospital doctor, community nursing service, the Hospice Information Service at St Christopher's Hospice, London (address at end of chapter), British Association of Cancer United Patients (BACUP), CancerLink or local self-help group.

The Hospice Information Service publishes a *Directory of Hospice Services* listing more than 200 hospices and home-care teams in the UK and Southern Ireland, including the names of the medical director, social worker and nursing officer of the units.

AREN'T THEY VERY DEPRESSING?

A glance at a hospice should dispel any fears about the workhouse. Many are purpose-built and all are designed to be relaxed, easy on the eye and comfortable. Several have landscaped gardens, cheerful day rooms and kitchens and sitting rooms for relatives.

Deaths are frequent in hospices but the depressing effect this might have on residents and visitors is offset by the benefits of a peaceful, secure environment, maintained by people who have chosen to specialize in this sort of care.

If you are unsure about a partner or relative going into a hospice ask if you can visit first. Staff should be happy to put your mind at rest. Families often arrive too distressed to speak and finish the visit by asking when the person can be admitted.

STAYING AT HOME

Although there is no definitive research on the subject it is widely assumed that, given the choice, most people would want to spend their last days at home. Familiar surroundings give a sense of security and lessen any possible fear or loneliness. By staying at home the sick person can maintain a certain control over their care, almost to the end, it is argued.

And there is no doubt that home care for people with advanced cancer can work well, giving the sick person a certain independence and the carer, and the family if any, a feeling of having done their best with good support from local medical services.

Given a willing GP who is up to date with pain-relief tech-niques and an efficient district nurse, possibly backed up by a specialist, such as a Macmillan nurse, there is no question that people can be well cared for at home, even when living alone. But looking after someone with advanced cancer is time consuming. The needs can vary from day to day, sometimes from hour to hour, and regular visits from the doctor or specialist nurse to fine-tune the drugs for pain relief and keep other symptoms under control are often required. Someone being looked after at home will benefit, in theory, from a 'multidisciplinary approach'. This means that several people will be involved: GP, district nurse, possibly a health visitor, specialist nurse and perhaps a few others besides.

That can work well and it often boosts the sick person's morale to be attended by several professionals. But in some cases the patient, and especially the carer, may find themselves longing for one familiar, fairly constant face who could deal with the problem *now*. Where communication is less than perfect messages may not be responded to immediately and relatives may be left wondering where to turn. Traffic jams and the demands of a large case-load may prevent people from turning up when they are expected, heightening the anxiety of the sick person and whoever is looking after them.

Your GP may be reluctant to take on the commitment home care involves, because of lack of time, desire or expertise. The average GP with a list of 2000 patients would normally see only five people a year dying at home – not enough, some specialists feel, to keep them experienced and up to date with advances in care. With the best will in the world some conscientious GPs feel that they are simply unable to give the dying the time they deserve and that a hospice or hospital would provide better care. And GPs who are regularly unavailable at nights and weekends, turning their calls over to a deputizing service, are unlikely to want to give families the sort of support they are looking for.

This is not to minimize the potentials of home care, which are enormous, but to encourage realistic consideration of the factors involved. However wide the range of professional advice it is likely to be the partner or family who bear the brunt of 24-hour care. And although standards have improved, with growing interest in the dying, home care has also been severely criticized. A study by cancer care specialist Professor Eric Wilkes, published in 1984, described the quality of life of people nursed at home as 'poor or very poor' in 44 per cent of cases. GPs were criticized by relatives for lack of interest, and failure to provide explanations or to examine the patient properly. Difficulties in getting medical help at night, except from a deputizing doctor who didn't know the case, and delays of up to eight weeks in obtaining aids such as incontinence pads caused anxiety.

And, it seems, some GPs cheerfully make light of what is involved in home care. 'I give them a bottle of morphine and tell them to get on with it,' was one GP's answer for people with cancer pain, according to a letter in the *British Medical Journal.* This blithely confident practitioner added that he never gave instructions on how often the patients should take the drug: 'They take it when they feel they need it.'

HOME CARE – WHO'S WHO?

The following is a brief guide to the people who are most likely to be involved in looking after someone with cancer at home, and their usual roles.

GENERAL PRACTITIONER

Ideally the GP should be both the lynch pin and instigator of home care, familiar with the patient, and family, if any, and local nursing and social services. When it is clear someone is becoming increasingly dependent it is up to the GP to assess the overall needs for medical and nursing care and to mobilize the relevant help. Once home care is underway, involving a range of staff, the person with cancer is likely to see more of the district nurse than the GP. But overall responsibility for the patient at home always lies with the GP, who is also responsible for prescribing any drugs required. The GP is also usually responsible for arranging admission to a hospital or hospice, where necessary.

DISTRICT NURSES

District nurses, or community nurses as they are now known, do not provide constant care in the hospital sense of the term but can pay regular visits to give injections or bed baths or to help with bathing, bowel and catheter care and changes of dressings. In some cases they can visit up to three times a day. They can also arrange for practical aids such as incontinence pads, bed rests, commodes, ramps, handrails, a raised lavatory seat, and a hospital bed to be delivered to the home free.

It is up to the district nurse, often in conjunction with a Macmillan nurse, to monitor the person's medication and response to drugs and to inform the GP when changes seem necessary.

MACMILLAN NURSES

There are more than 300 Macmillan nurses working in the community, alongside GPs, social workers, district nurses and consultants, any of whom may refer a patient to them.

Macmillan nurses have undergone a six-weeks' specialist training in symptom and pain control, counselling and care of the dying. They do not normally provide continuous day-to-day home nursing, in the sense of baths and bowel care. But they make regular visits to monitor the person's drug regime and can assist district nurses in setting up syringe drivers or pumps which allow drugs to be administered automatically. They are particularly aware of the emotional problems cancer brings and often spend up to an hour on a home visit, paying attention to the welfare of the carer, of the rest of the family, as well as of the person with cancer.

Many Macmillan nurses are attached to hospices and continuing care units and, in conjunction with the GP, can arrange admission. Nurses, who operate in teams of two or more, make at least one follow-up visit after a death and some run bereavement groups.

Macmillan nurses are not available to every patient with cancer at home by any means. More than a quarter of Britain's health districts are still without Macmillan teams. But Cancer Relief, which sets up the teams and provides the initial running costs, which are then taken on by the NHS, aims to cover the whole country within a couple of years. The service is free.

MARIE CURIE NURSES

The Marie Curie Memorial Foundation (MCMF) has nurses working in most areas of the country who will give day or night cover in the home. The service is free to the patient, and is funded by the MCMF and the local health authority. The main demand of the service is for night nursing so that the main carer can get some rest.

To find out if there is a scheme in your area ring your local community nursing officer (listed under the district health authority) or the MCMF. The MCMF produces a series of leaflets on whom to contact in each health region to obtain day or night nursing at home for someone with cancer. Contact with the local service can also be made through the patient's GP, district nurse or health visitor.

SOCIAL WORKER

Social workers can advise on welfare and charitable benefits, claiming them on clients' behalf if necessary, as well as arranging home helps, Meals on Wheels, housing and special holidays. Where there are children who need to be looked after he or she can arrange care assistants. They also play a general counselling role and may act as mediators in family disputes.

You can contact a social worker through your doctor, district nurse or local authority social services department.

HEALTH VISITOR

The health visitor is particularly likely to take part in home care when young children are involved, and can arrange sitters if parents are absent for any reason. She can also arrange the delivery of equipment to the home, give general and bereavement counselling, and liaise with other services. She can also advise on local volunteer schemes able to help.

OCCUPATIONAL THERAPIST

Domiciliary occupational therapists are concerned with maintaining the person's comfort and independence at home. After an initial assessment visit she or he will be able to arrange for aids such as lavatory frames, handrails or a wheel chair to be delivered. The occupational therapist can also arrange for minor adaptations such as door widening or safety rails in bathrooms.

When people experience difficulty dressing or undressing the occupational therapist may be able to suggest adaptations to clothing and have the alterations carried out.

PHYSIOTHERAPIST

Domiciliary physiotherapists are generally brought in by the GP or district nurse. The physiotherapist can help keep someone mobile, contribute towards the relief of pain and help keep the lungs clear. Referral is usually through the district nurse, health visitor or GP.

HOME HELPS

Provision of home helps varies in different parts of the country, with some districts providing no service at all. To find out about local arrangements contact your local social services department, social worker, district nurse or GP. Where no alternative exists Cancer Relief will sometimes meet the cost of a private home help.

VOLUNTEERS AND HELPERS

Anyone looking after a sick person at home will need time out – even if only to do the shopping, go to the post office, visit the hairdresser or simply go for a walk. The GP, district nurse, or citizens advice bureau should know what help is available locally.

Some general practices now have patients' associations which organize volunteers to assist patients in any way they can, whether that is collecting and delivering prescriptions, arranging transport or sitting with someone so that the person looking after them can go out.

The Red Cross has a branch in every county and some 10 000 volunteers across the UK. Volunteers can help the housebound in a variety of ways, including shopping, posting letters and changing library books. The Red Cross also runs short courses for those looking after the dying at home. Local branches are listed in the telephone directory.

The Association of Carers has more than 250 groups, some of which provide sit-in services to give the regular carer a break. The Association keeps a list of groups and, even if your local one does not organize a volunteer attendant, scheme members are likely to know what is available.

Liverpool has had a volunteer scheme specifically for the support of people dying at home and their carers since 1983. The Liverpool Personal Service Society has more than twenty volunteers visiting some thirty homes to provide respite for the family and company for the sick person. Volunteers arrange transport, help with chores, assist with funeral arrangements if required and visit relatives after the death.

Similar schemes operate in other areas, although not neces- sarily restricted to the needs of the dying. The Lockwood Care Attendant Service, operating in Hackney, East London, for ex- ample, is a seven-days-a-week service catering to a variety of needs. Although not normally able to provide sitters for people in the very last stages of illness, the scheme supplies escorts for people going to hospital and someone to look after the children while a parent is out. The attendants often help out while other services such as Meals on Wheels and home helps are being arranged.

GENERAL HELP ON AIDS AND EQUIPMENT

The Disabled Living Foundation runs an information service dealing with more than 20 000 inquiries a year. It has specialist advisers on incontinence and clothing and has occupational thera- pists and physiotherapists who can give personal advice on aids and equipment. An appointment is necessary for individual con- sultations. The exhibition in its show-rooms in West London (address at end of chapter) features more than 1000 pieces of equipment, which can be demonstrated, from special cutlery to walking aids, bathroom supplies and wheel chairs.

POINTS TO REMEMBER WHEN PLANNING HOME CARE

Ideally any discussion of care should involve the GP, family and person being looked after so that a realistic plan can be drawn up which leaves relatives in no doubt about what support they can count on. The doctor should make clear what sort of help can be brought in to the home and what this will mean in terms of hours, frequency and reliability. The points outlined below should be covered.

Day care

- Who will be the principal carer? Wife, husband, daughter, son, other relative, friend? Will they be there all day or out part of the time because of work and collecting children from school?
- What times of day is the carer likely to be out? Can anyone else, such as a daughter, neighbour or friend, cover that time? Every day, twice a week, occasionally?
- Who can provide a sitting service for the times the family cannot cover? Who will arrange this – GP, social worker, district nurse?
- Who will provide help with dressing and bathing if required? And how often?
- Who will give injections, if needed?
- How often will the GP visit? Once a week, every day, or only on request?
- If help or advice is needed urgently how can the GP be contacted? Where can you leave an urgent message?
- Is a home help necessary? If so, how many times a week is this possible? Is there a charge? How soon can one be fixed?
- If the person being looked after is incontinent, or likely to become so, is there a laundry service? How often does it collect.
- Are Macmillan nurses available locally? How much time and care will they be able to give?

Night care

- If the person being looked after needs attention several times during the night, or more or less constantly, is there anyone who can help, besides the carer? Can a relative or friend spend the night once or twice a week?
- Will night nursing be needed and if so who will provide this? The Marie Curie service? A hospice home-care team? A private agency nurse? If the latter, can help be provided towards the cost? By Cancer Relief, or a provident association such as British United Provident Association (BUPA) if the person is covered?
- Who should the relative/family/carer/patient telephone in case of emergency?
- Is there always someone who can give advice and make a visit if necessary? GP? Home-care team?

Home comforts

Home care is bound to have its ups and downs, but an early assessment of day-to-day activities can simplify life both for the person being looked after and for the carer. The following points are worth considering:

- Is the person as comfortable as possible? In bed? Sitting up in a chair (a rubber ring on the chair may help)? Moving around the home?
- If not, a hospital bed, high armchair and walking frame, borrowed from the district nursing service, could make all the difference.
- If the bedroom and lavatory are a long way apart, or on different floors, it may be sensible to move the sick person nearer, even into the sitting room if needs be.
- For someone confined to bed a ripple mattress to prevent pressure sores, or a sheepskin (on loan from the district nursing service) and a bed table of the correct height, can improve life considerably.
- Is the home warm/cool enough for the sick person's comfort? Fans and heaters may be available on loan through social services or the district nurse or, in cases of hardship, may be bought with a grant from Cancer Relief, which also gives help towards heating costs and extra bedding.

● Telephone: looking after someone in need of more or less constant attention can be nerve-racking if you cannot reach other
people quickly. Apart from the need to summon help, a telephone
will help the housebound person keep in touch and is more or
less essential where close relatives are living abroad, or in other
parts of the country. If social services will not pay for one to be
installed, Cancer Relief can help.

Knowing where to turn

Nobody is immune from exhaustion, however great the love
and commitment to the person they are looking after. Disturbed
nights and distress at a loved one's frailty can make you very tired
indeed. But finding out, early on, what sort of back-up support is
available, should you need it, can give peace of mind. Is a bed
available in the local hospice, continuing care unit or hospital if
you feel you can't go on or need a break? You may feel able, and
happy, to cope throughout, but it is always reassuring to know
what help is available, should the need arise.

After hospital treatment for cancer of the oesophagus, 46-
year-old Sid Harvey was adamant he wanted to stay at home for
the rest of his life. His wife, Jean, was well supported by relatives
willing to help with cooking and shopping. But she was worried
about being able to keep him comfortable.

The district nurse and consultant suggested the Macmillan
home-care team based at a community clinic in Ipswich. The three
nurses brought his pain under control and taught her how to give
injections – so that she was able to give him his drugs every three
hours. 'I was a bit anxious about it at first but it was such a relief
not to have to worry about the pain coming back all the time,' she
recalls.

Sid enjoyed the nurses' visits and was happy to let them help
him. 'He was a barber and never normally let anyone touch his
hair. But he was quite happy for one of the nurses to cut it while he
gave instructions.' The nurses helped sell his van, agreeing the final
price with him.

During the ten weeks he was at home in bed Sid put his
affairs in order and made the arrangements for his funeral. 'He
always liked to be in charge and I'm happy he kept that feeling

right up to his death,' says Jean. 'People think looking after someone who is dying will be depressing, but it wasn't. There was a lot of warmth and humour in the last days and we talked a lot. It was quite smooth and happy.'

Jean valued the emotional support of the home-care team as much as their practical help. 'You feel they are interested in you as well as the patient and that's very helpful. It's someone for yourself.' After his death Jean kept in touch with the team and attended their bereavement group.

USEFUL ADDRESSES

Hospice Information Service
St Christopher's Hospice
51–59 Lawrie Park Road
London SE26 6DZ
Tel: 01-778 1240

Macmillan Services
National Society for Cancer
Relief
Anchor House
15/19 Britten Street
London SW3 3TZ
Tel: 01-351 7811

Marie Curie Memorial Foundation
28 Belgrave Square
London SW1X 8QG
Tel: 01-235 3325

Association of Carers
First Floor
21–23 New Road
Chatham
Kent ME4 4QJ
Tel: 0634 813981

Sue Ryder Homes
Cavendish
Suffolk CO10 8AY
Tel: 0787 280252

Disabled Living Foundation
380/384 Harrow Road
London W9 2HU
Tel: 01-289 6111

The British Red Cross Society
9 Grosvenor Crescent
London SW1X 7EJ
Tel: 01-235 5454

Liverpool Personal Service
Society
34 Stanley Street
Liverpool L1 6AN
Tel: 051-236 5255

Lockwood Care Attendant
Service
St Leonard's Hospital
Nuttall Street
Hackney
London N1 5LZ
Tel: 01-739 9277

Chapter Twelve

WILL LIFE EVER BE THE SAME?

'We think of ourselves as living with cancer, not dying from it.' (Beth Howard, founder of Coping with Cancer Nottingham, seven years after her ovarian cancer was diagnosed)

'People who have chronic cancer continue to raise their children, work, eat in restaurants, go to movies, love and make love, and travel. The experience of cancer has, of course changed us. We have had to come to grips with our mortality, and are stronger for that. We have had to determine our priorities and focus our energies accordingly. But having stared death in the face, we have an infinitely deeper understanding of life.' (Jory Graham in *In The Company of Others*)

'Life's very different and much more focused than before. I don't get upset by traffic jams or office politics and family and friends have become much more important.' (Dr Vicky Clement-Jones, British Association of Cancer United Patients)

'I still want to be rich – stinking rich – but I think I've got ambition in its proper place now.' (George Cohen, former World Cup footballer)

'Progress in treatment is not enough. People must be restored to a full emotional life as well.' (Professor Tim McElwain, Head of Medicine, Royal Marsden Hospital)

Will life ever be the same again? Yes and no. Few major experiences, by definition, can leave us completely unchanged in terms of outlook, understanding and disposition, and cancer is no exception. It is, after all, a reminder of mortality and frailty, however treatable the form it takes. But thousands do live with cancer, or the possibility of cancer recurring, without being condemned to a half-life, as the accounts in this chapter show.

And without sounding false many report life being sharper and more focused as a result of their illness and the reassessment involved. Some therapists talk of cancer as a transformational illness and many people find it triggers a complete review of their lives and priorities. Some people continue pretty much as before, but others, as one woman described it, 'use cancer as a cue for a complete clear out', examining their relationships and values.

On a more basic level cancer may demand the postponement or reshaping of long-term plans – for a change of job, a bigger mortgage or an addition to the family. But it need not mean the abandonment of all goals and ambition, providing these are pursued with flexibility and a certain preparedness for setbacks. The life will not be identical to the one you had before, but it can be whole.

WILL THERE ALWAYS BE SOMETHING HANG-ING OVER ME?

Cancer is still associated with imminent death in many people's minds. And when first told they have cancer people are often preoccupied by a feeling they are about to die, whatever the facts about their individual case and type of cancer. The negative connotations of the disease frequently override any reassurances given in the early consultations.

But survival rates have improved markedly during this century. In 1900 less than 20 per cent of people with cancer were cured. Now it is more than 40 per cent for all cancers taken together, with higher rates for Hodgkin's disease and younger age-groups.

Some people are cured of cancer in the sense that they go on to live a normal lifespan and die from something else. And thousands of others have their symptoms controlled in a way which enables them to continue with normal life.

Doctors are reluctant to talk of cure because cancer can recur after many symptom-free years. But some people not only survive several recurrences but also maintain an active life between episodes of illness and treatment.

But some uncertainty about the future is felt by most people who have, or have had, cancer. It is likely to be most intense immediately after diagnosis, on the completion of treatment and in the days preceding check-ups, and gradually lessens with the passage of time. It is unusual for people to remain extremely anxious for more than two years after a diagnosis of cancer where treatment appears to have been successful.

None the less, everyone found to have cancer must come to terms with the fact that they have a life-threatening, often unpredictable disease, which may disrupt their plans and expectations. Many find it helpful, particularly just after diagnosis and during the early days of treatment, consciously to take things one day at a time without worrying about the long-term outlook. This approach is particularly appropriate when you are very anxious and below par physically. At times of great strain it can be helpful to remind yourself that nobody can live more than a day at a time. People who manage to do this find that anxiety lessens and general confidence increases as they start to return to normal life.

Of course people with cancer must take on board the possibility that they may one day die from it. But that does not mean that the thought dominates their life and outlook, or that it somehow undermines their commitment and enjoyment. The best adjusted often make a firm decision to live as fully as possible and not to let doubts about the future hamper enjoyment of the present. They feel able, and eager, to control the quality of day-to-day life without worrying what hurdles may appear in the future.

HOW TO HELP YOURSELF

There is a growing realization that psychological support for people with cancer is often woefully inadequate both at the time of diagnosis and later on. Specialist units have recently been set up at the Royal Marsden Hospital, London, and the Christie Hospital, Manchester, to look at the difficulties people with cancer face and to establish appropriate support schemes which, it is hoped, will be adopted by general hospitals.

Meanwhile there is general agreement that people can help themselves adjust to living with cancer through positive thinking and an assertive attitude towards life and enjoyment. While it has yet to be proved that this approach actually prolongs life there is no doubt that it improves morale, giving people a feeling of being in control of their own lives.

Specialists say that no one should accept persistent depression or a general feeling of colourlessness as inevitable side-effects of cancer. There are ways of coping with general depression and with particular causes of stress such as recurrences and check-ups.

DEPRESSION: WHEN TO GET HELP

About one in four people with cancer suffer serious emotional disturbance as a result of their illness and are in need of specialist help. Psychiatrists specializing in helping people with cancer find that improvements in morale are often very rapid once difficulties are uncovered. But it is important that those having great difficulties should seek help early on and not expect a stiff upper lip to see them through. Partners and relatives should also encourage someone who continues to be very upset to seek help.

What are the signs that someone needs help? Intense reactions to the diagnosis of cancer are to be expected, but if any of the following persist for more than three or four weeks it may be an indication that extra help is needed: crying, sleeplessness, difficulty in concentrating, loss of interest, lack of appetite, irritability, withdrawal, brittleness, or getting annoyed for no reason. If someone seems stuck in depression and their mood does not lift, however much support and understanding is offered, that is a clear indication that they need specialist help.

Report such reactions to your G P or hospital doctor and ask what can be done. You may be referred to a psychiatrist or specialist nurse. Studies have shown that doctors tend to concentrate on physical problems when asking people with cancer about their health. So it will very likely be up to you to bring up emotional problems and make sure that help is given.

CHECK-UPS

Check-ups are often stressful for anyone who has, or has had, cancer and anxiety is likely to increase in the days leading up to them. Obviously the worry is likely to be reduced with time and with 'clear' checks. But it is common to feel some apprehension as you return to the hospital which may have upsetting associations, reminding you of the uncertainty you felt at the time of diagnosis and during treatment.

It can help your peace of mind to discuss check-ups with your doctor early on, to clarify what tests you will have, what they can establish and why a particular interval has been chosen. If you have been told to return every three months after treatment for breast cancer, while your friend who has had the same treatment has been told she will have check-ups at six-month intervals, that does not automatically mean that you are considered to be at greater risk of a recurrence. Her surgeon may simply have a policy of seeing everyone at six-month intervals while yours favours three-month.

Discussing follow-ups before the end of your treatment can save a lot of worry and it may be possible to 'negotiate' with your doctor for an arrangement you feel at ease with.

There is no doubt that some people draw valuable reassurance from regular check-ups, so much so that hospitals are still seeing people who were successfully treated twenty years ago and more. But for others check-ups cause such anxiety that the drawbacks seem to outweigh the benefits. And such people might find it easier to return only when worried about a particular symptom or a marked deterioration. Some doctors go so far as to say that fixed interval check-ups are unnecessary, serving only to increase anxiety, and that people sense any change which needs investigation and will report this of their own accord.

You may also find it helpful to review the way you are being followed up with your doctor each year. As time goes on you may feel happy to increase the intervals between check-ups. Do not simply go along with the set policy without knowing how that relates to your individual needs. And make sure that the results are explained in a way which tells you all you want to know. Do not be content with 'everything seems to be under control' or 'you seem to have a little bit of the old trouble' unless you are quite happy to leave things to your doctor.

RECURRENCES

You have coped with treatment, recovered from the side-effects, returned to normal life and are beginning to feel cancer is really behind you. Then, months or years later you find it has come back. Whether fighters or deniers, most people who have experienced recurrences agree that this was their all-time low and that coping a second or third time around requires a great deal of determination.

If you were assertive facing the disease first time around and have thought of yourself conquering cancer you may look on a recurrence as a kind of failure. At such times it may be helpful to remind yourself that nobody has established a sure-fire way of avoiding recurrences, so you should not blame yourself for what you see as failure to think positively; change your diet or whatever.

Rather than thinking that you have lost a major battle in a continuing war against cancer it may be helpful to look on a recurrence as an isolated episode and something you will cope with, just as before you coped with the original diagnosis and treatment.

Life can go on after one or more recurrences, as two accounts at the end of the chapter explain.

THE PLEASURE PRINCIPLE

What do you most enjoy doing, visitors to the Bristol Cancer Help Centre are regularly asked. Many cannot answer and a significant number say they feel guilty thinking about themselves in such a direct way. But it is an important question. Everyone needs pleasure to brighten their lives and to lighten the load of humdrum tasks. Real enjoyment gives relaxation, renewal and a sense of being at ease with ourselves and the world. Yet a surprising number of people either never discover what gives them joy or are permanently postponing pleasure, until they have tidied the house, redecorated, taken the exam, got a better job, cleared out the attic or whatever. It is as if enjoyment had to be earned and some people never feel they have acquired enough points.

Of course it is important to have goals and the carrot-and-stick approach does help some people through their tasks and towards the desired object. But at the same time we have only one chance to enjoy today and joyless lives soon lose their savour.

So if enjoying yourself is something you have never really thought about, give it some consideration and make sure that each week, preferably each day, includes something that makes you feel good. It does not have to be worthy or constructive but should give you a definite feeling of pleasure and well-being. Gardening, swimming, walking, painting, listening to appealing music or telephoning a friend – the activity need not be elaborate or expensive but should lift your mood and provide a break from everyday concerns. Most people believe they are less likely to get ill when they are relaxed and happy. And some therapists believe that pleasure actually boosts the immune system. Whether or not this is true, people getting over cancer frequently remark on how much better they feel once they have thought about what brings them pleasure and have deliberately made time for enjoyment.

Cancer may at times restrict your mobility and reduce your energy, but that is no reason to suspend your appetite for entertainment and diversion.

It is a mistake to assume that cancer will automatically limit any of your capacities and particularly that for enjoyment. Illness and treatment may take you out of the social stream occasionally, but should not do so permanently.

*

Dame Mary Donaldson, London's first woman Lord Mayor, was 53 when she found a lump in her breast and underwent a mastectomy. Another lump, four years later, led to a second mastectomy. Each time she took only a few weeks off before returning to a busy public life and her favourite sports: sailing, swimming and skiing. Eight years on she feels 'absolutely fit' and is only prepared to talk about her illness to encourage others about life after cancer.

A former chairman of the Women's National Cancer Control Campaign, she has a long-standing interest in the disease stretching back to her wartime nursing days at the Middlesex Hospital.

'When I first discovered it was cancer, I was very angry and felt, why me? I was very busy and resentful of the interruption. At the time of the first operation I was wondering whether to stand as an Alderman and had many commitments. So I had to get back into the swing and I think that was helpful. If you've got to get out and do something it's so much easier.

'When it recurred I was very frightened, but also relieved to find the lump was primary and not a secondary from the original cancer. I had the operation in January and was skiing in April.

'Now I go for check-ups every six months but I don't feel anything hanging over me. I haven't changed my outlook and my life is planned two to three years ahead, just as it always was. It's a very intensive life and I'm going out all day.

'But there's slight resentment that this thing will always be with me. Every time I get a pain anywhere which lasts more than a few days I wonder whether it's a secondary, and, more annoying, I can't even have a sore throat without other people suspecting the worst. Before I went in for the mayoralty people used to come up to me and ask "Are you sure you will not find the year too exhausting?" I found that very annoying. You are rather labelled once you've had cancer.

'My lowest times were just after I came out of hospital but I didn't feel diminished or particularly disfigured. I nursed the men from Dunkirk and the loss of a breast seemed very minor compared with the mutilations I saw then.

'But I do think counselling is important and having access to someone who has been through the same thing. Someone you can ring up and talk to so there isn't that awful lonely gap when you get home. My husband found a judge's wife who had had the same operation who came to visit me in hospital. It was very encouraging.

'There are still problems, such as communal changing rooms.

I rush off to find a loo when everyone is stripping off. And I sometimes yearn for really glamorous swim-suits. But on the whole I feel very lucky. I am very happily married and have a close family and cancer did not change that at all. The treatment has been successful to all intents and purposes and cancer never stopped me from doing anything I wanted to. . . .'

*

Writer and photographer Francis Goodman was 65 when he was told he must have his bladder removed, having undergone radiotherapy six years earlier.

'At the time I was feeling wonderful and it came as quite a shock. I had been going for check-ups and a cystoscopy every three months but felt completely well.

'Just before the operation I went on assignment to the South of France and crossing the Italian border I wondered whether I would ever do that again. I did feel a bit sad but then I thought I'd had a good life, whatever was to happen. And I finished my article before going into hospital. The operation involved making a hole in the wall of the abdomen where urine would be collected in a disposable plastic pouch.

'I didn't know what to expect after the operation and would have liked a lot more information. I thought I would have some sort of bicycle valve coming out of my stomach on to which I would screw a kind of bag. Just before the operation they did show me the sort of bag I was to have but I didn't know how to cope. And after the operation I was so whacked I was incapable of constructive thought. After five weeks in hospital and two in a convalescent home I was still very tired and still didn't know how to put on the bag securely. I hadn't been properly taught and didn't even know how to have a bath. For three months I was totally at a loss.

'Back at home I got completely desperate one day and rang up the Ileostomy Association who were very informative and told me about the stoma care service at the Royal Marsden Hospital. When I rang the hospital the stoma care nurse was away but they sent round two district nurses who were very helpful.

'Later on I had a three-hour talk with the stoma care nurse at the Marsden and we went through everything. It was marvellous. The Marsden really helped me feel independent again. My passing-out parade as I call it was changing the bag alone in Harrods' gents.

'The nurse told me that my real freedom would come when I started doing what I loved. And she was proved completely right. One day the *Daily Telegraph* rang and asked me to do two articles on cycle touring and I felt as if I had been thrown a lifeline. That led to other assignments and now I go abroad six or seven times a year. At 74 I'm doing what I've always wanted to do – writing and travelling. And I've never been more content.

'But just after the operation I felt extremely depressed. I think it was about six months before my emotions stabilized. I used to look at pictures in the paper and think they are whole people, I no longer am. I felt that I no longer belonged to the world and that nothing could ever be of interest again. But that passed completely.

'I knew I was getting into life again when I took myself off to buy a new dressing-gown. At first I thought I would never enjoy anything frivolous again.

'Now I am totally adjusted and completely fulfilled in my work. Of course if you could choose you would rather not have a bag, just as you would prefer not to have false teeth. But I never think about having had cancer. I think it's very important that you get on with life and don't get stuck. My advice to anyone would be get as much information as possible, learn to cope and don't look back. I'm not courageous, I'm a bit of a rabbit really. But finding I could cope gave me an extra strength.'

*

George Cohen, aged 47, a member of the England football team which won the World Cup in 1966, now working as a builder and property developer, was 36 when he started to feel lethargic and depressed and developed severe diarrhoea. An exploratory operation revealed cancer of the rectum and part of his colon was removed. After ten weeks in hospital he made a complete recovery and returned to a normal life. But 18 months later he had a recurrence and was given a colostomy.

'I was pleased the doctors were so straightforward and felt

"right let's get on with it". I was never one to be afraid of what people might tell you. After all if you're going to die, you'll die anyway whether they tell you or not.

'I had no problems with the colostomy. You've got to be positive, it's going to be with you for the rest of your life. And the specialist nurse was wonderful. She suggested my wife should see it right away. There were some restrictions such as not being able to have a rough and tumble with the kids when they were young. But I eat and drink what I want.'

A year after the colostomy operation he became ill again and his left foot became swollen. The doctor said the growth had spread to his back and was pressing on a nerve. He could not work and had to be taken by ambulance to hospital every day for six weeks' radiotherapy. He was also having twice-daily injections for the pain from a district nurse.

'I was worried but never thought I was going to die. And my wife Daphne's positive attitude was very helpful. I once felt I didn't care what happened and she gave me a good rollicking. Gradually you do pick yourself up and start to think positively again. . . . It was a recession and I lost a huge amount of money but after six months I could walk again and got back to work. I think the discipline of my football days and general fitness helped.

'When I first heard it was cancer I wanted to scream my head off and felt terribly out of breath. But when I told my wife she put her arms around me and just said "When do you go to the hospital?" She took it as something we had to face together.

'Initially we didn't tell the kids it was cancer, but I showed them the colostomy right at the beginning so they'd know what I was coping with. They took it in a very matter of fact way.

'At first I wondered in a macho way what I would look like in bed with my wife with this bag hanging down. And at times I do get depressed about the colostomy. You look at yourself in the mirror and think "God, look at that" and remember back to what you were – a very fit person.

'It's never stopped me from doing anything I wanted and I lead a completely normal life. But cancer has changed my attitudes. I get up at six, go into the garden and think how wonderful it is to be alive. Life is certainly more precious and I get very annoyed at people who moan or throw their lives away with drugs.

'I don't believe cancer is anything to hide. Of course I know I may die from it but at least I can live with the right sort of attitude now.

'I always want to be stinking rich but think that's because I'm fairly generous and want to give as much as possible to those I love.

'Once you've had cancer there's always the thought in the back of your mind that it could come back. That is when I remind myself that I've got over it three times and could probably get over it a fourth – I would just batten down the hatches again and have a go. That seems to make the cloud disappear.'

*

Viscount Tonypandy, formerly George Thomas, Speaker of the House of Commons, was 74 when he developed cancer of the larynx in 1984. After six weeks' radiotherapy he took up his normal life again, undertaking regular speaking engagements.

'They told me the chance of a cure was high and I felt then that I was home and dry. I never felt this is the end. I have had a very full life and am not afraid of death, but I do like it down here. My faith made a big difference to me.

'During the treatment my spirits were quite high but afterwards I did feel a bit low for a time and sometimes had difficulty swallowing. Now I have a very enjoyable, crowded life. I can't speak for more than about twelve minutes, because I get hoarse and I've had to slow down a bit. But at my age that might have happened anyway.

'I never like to say I'm in the clear but I feel well and confident enough about the future to accept engagements two years ahead. I don't dwell on having had cancer but it has made me appreciate each day more, and deepened my faith.

'I never thought of not telling anyone about it, and I think the terrible fear we've had about the word cancer needs blowing away. Even when it's not curable doctors can prolong life and make it bearable.

'I could see from the sad look in their eyes some people

thought I was written off. But I have never had so many invitations
to speak. It simply isn't true that you are finished once you have cancer. And I think we have a duty to encourage each other. I met with a lot of affection and that certainly helped.

'My only regret is that I can't sing hymns any more. I used to love that.'

Chapter Thirteen

LOOKING TO THE FUTURE

WHAT HAS BEEN ACHIEVED SO FAR?

In the last decade US politicians coined the slogan 'Let's beat cancer in the 70s'. Having put man on the moon in the 1960s, some thought that if you poured enough money into cancer research you were sure to come up with an answer. More than fifteen years of cancer charities topping the league table of donations for medical research on both sides of the Atlantic has not brought 'the answer'. The money has not been wasted; there has been a major leap forward in the understanding of what turns a normal cell into a cancer cell. The value of screening for some tumours, such as cervical and breast cancer, has been recognized. The message about the danger of cigarettes leading to lung cancer has at last been getting through – at least to male smokers. Developments in scanning equipment and in laboratory tests have meant that some cancers are being diagnosed earlier so that there is a greater chance of successful treatment.

The way in which cancer is treated has become much more precise; many of the drugs in current use have been around for twenty, even thirty, years. But doctors have become much more adept at using them. Higher doses are possible now that there are better facilities to cope with the side-effects of treatment; combinations of drugs have frequently proved more effective than single drugs on their own.

Thanks to the more detailed pictures obtainable through scanning techniques, courses of radiotherapy can be planned much more precisely. Not only does this ensure that the tumour receives the maximum possible dose, it also helps reduce the risk of damage to surrounding tissue. Advances in diagnosis have also enabled surgeons to be much more precise in the way they remove tumours.

Guided by accurate X-rays they can remove tumours too small to be seen with the naked eye. Calcium deposits picked up on an X-ray may be the only sign of the beginnings of breast cancer, for example, but surgeons can remove the affected tissue before a tumour has a chance to develop.

Perhaps as significant as the advances in diagnosis and treatment of cancer has been the growing realization that quality of life is as important as quantity of life to someone with cancer. People are demanding to know more about their disease, the options for treatment and how these can be made more acceptable. Side-effects do not have to be worse than the disease and frequently they can be prevented. People can help themselves and each other, as the expanding network of self-help and support groups has shown. In 1986 the Cancer Research Campaign set up two research groups to find ways of measuring emotional distress in people with cancer and to develop treatment for relieving it.

So far, the real success stories in cancer have been limited. But 'cure' is now a word which is commonly used in many childhood cancers, Hodgkin's lymphoma and leukaemia, and in the rarer adult genital tumours – testicular and choriocarcinoma. In twenty years the cure rate for testicular teratoma has risen from around 50 per cent, achieved almost solely with surgery in men whose tumours had not spread, to over 90 per cent, and including even quite advanced cancers, thanks to the introduction of better drugs. At least two-thirds of people with Hodgkin's disease can now expect to survive, compared with only 30 per cent in 1965. And nearly all women who get choriocarcinoma are now cured, compared with virtually no one thirty years ago.

Having achieved such successes with some relatively uncommon cancers the emphasis must now be on more effective treatment for the big three killers: lung cancer, which accounts for 40 per cent of all cancer deaths, breast cancer and bowel cancer. So what are scientists doing in their search for better treatment of these cancers? And will it be possible ever to prevent cancer and reduce the need for cure?

WHERE DO WE GO FROM HERE?

SCREENING

Cervical cancer lends itself to screening. From the normal, healthy cells at the 'white' end of the spectrum to the advanced spreading cancer at the 'black' end there are many shades of 'grey' which can be picked up and monitored by regular smear tests. Some of the earliest changes may mean nothing; they do not even fall into the 'pre-malignant' group and they may well revert to normal by the time of the next smear. But as evidence grows that a high proportion of abnormal cervical cells contain evidence of the wart papilloma virus so women must demand more frequent smears to pick up the first signs of infection. Often all that is needed is a 'wait and see' approach. Smears can be taken every three or six months after the first slightly abnormal test. If the cells revert to normal no further treatment is needed. But, if they progress, early treatment can remove the unhealthy tissue before there is any chance of an invasive cancer.

The screening service in the UK remains a shambles and even where women are given regular cervical smears the laboratories are frequently so weighed down with requests that there are long delays in getting results. Hopefully it is just a matter of time before a proper, nationwide, computerized service is set up. The scientific case for regular cervical screening is proven.

Breast cancer

Results are expected at any time from a major study involving nearly a quarter of a million women to see if regular breast X-rays (mammography) can pick up early breast tumours. Other studies have already suggested that routine screening for breast cancer, especially for those at high risk, is worthwhile. Until now the emphasis has been on regular self-examination once a month for the first signs of any lumps and bumps. The problem with this is that by the time a lump can be felt it may be well advanced, whereas an X-ray can pick up the very earliest changes. Scientists are so optimistic that the screening study will show that X-rays are useful that the government has already been persuaded to set up a mammography programme for older women.

Bowel cancer

This is another type of cancer where screening may prove worthwhile. Most people with bowel tumours do notice some blood in their faeces but many others miss this early sign of the disease. However, it is possible to identify blood in faeces even when it is not visible to the naked eye. Clearly, it would not be feasible for people regularly to send a sample of faeces to a laboratory, but there are alternatives. Already one company has marketed a special type of toilet paper which changes colour in contact with small amounts of blood and it would be fairly easy for people to use this method at home. It seems likely that other simple methods may be developed which people could use at home. Then, if there was any doubt about the result they could be referred to hospital for further checks.

Skin cancer

An experimental educational programme was recently tested in western Scotland to increase awareness of malignant melanoma. This is the form of skin cancer most often linked to exposure to sunlight; if it is not picked up early it is frequently fatal. Many of these tumours start as harmless-looking moles or birthmarks. The most dangerous tumours are those which burrow downwards into the skin rather than spreading across the surface. The idea of an educational programme is to make people aware of the potential dangers of a mole or other mark which suddenly starts growing, changes shape or in some other way alters its appearance.

Other types of cancer

Unfortunately, there is no evidence that screening programmes could help pick up other types of cancer. The point about cervical, breast, bowel and skin cancers is that there is good evidence that if treated early the chances of cure are significantly improved. Each of these tumours either shows a well-defined visible series of pre-malignant changes or it is a slow-growing tumour or it occurs mainly in well-defined high-risk individuals. The same is not true of most other cancers.

MORE ACCURATE DIAGNOSIS

Ten years ago hospitals were trying to raise money for the £500 000 computerized body scanners which use X-rays to take pictures of thin cross-sectional 'slices' of the body instead of the conventional vertical X-rays. Because they combine dozens of X-rays into a single picture the results of these computerized axial tomogram (CAT or CT) scans are far more detailed than previous diagnostic techniques. The results can be further improved by using dyes injected into veins to produce a greater contrast between different types of tissue.

With a few notable exceptions most major hospitals now have access to CT scanners and a handful of hospitals have the new generation of scanners which do not use X-rays at all. Nuclear magnetic resonance (NMR) scanning uses a combination of powerful magnetic fields and radio waves to get remarkably detailed pictures of the body, frequently in areas where CT scanners are less good at getting pictures. But they are still under investigation and much of the work is still experimental. It seems likely that they will complement rather than supersede CT scanners.

Ultrasound scanners will also have a continuing role in cancer diagnosis. It is their small size and mobility which put them at an advantage for scans of specific areas, particularly in the abdomen. All but the smallest hospitals have one or more of these machines, though their effectiveness depends largely on the skill of the operator. Ultrasound scanners, like NMR, have the advantage of not using X-rays.

There is increasing use of radioactive isotopes for detection of tumours. These are injected into blood vessels and, as they disperse about the body, gamma cameras are used to photograph the radiation which is emitted and which distinguishes normal from cancerous tissue. Depending on the type of particle which is emitted, CT scanners and possibly NMR can be used together with the isotopes.

Research is currently underway to make this technique even more specific. Instead of allowing the radioactive isotope to find its own way to the tumour, doctors are attaching a sort of biological magnet which is attracted towards tumour cells. This new approach, being studied on only a few hundred patients at a handful of specialist centres around the world, has been made possible with the discovery that some types of tumour produce easily recognizable substances, called antigens.

In fact, all cells have antigens on their surfaces which help distinguish them from other cells. These antigens are generally made of protein and give the body its own special immune fingerprints. Each of us has a system of defence cells to protect us from intruders. This system, of which antibodies are the main fighting force, has a record of all its own antigens and does not attack them. Only if foreign antigens appear, be they invading microbes, badly matched blood transfusions or transplanted organs, do the protective antibodies come out and latch onto the foreign material.

Some cancer cells have antigens on their surface which are different from those on normal cells, but for some reason they are not recognized as abnormal and so are not destroyed by the immune system. Some of these antigens stay on the cells while others drop off and drift into the bloodstream where they can be measured. Two of the first of these tumour-associated antigens (TAA) to be recognized were human chorionic gonadotrophin (HCG) and carcinoembryonic antigen (CEA). Strictly speaking, HCG is a hormone which is produced during pregnancy. However, levels also rise in women with the placental tumour, choriocarcinoma. CEA is much more orthodox. It is a straightforward antigen found on the surface of cells in a number of different types of cancer, most notably bowel tumours and gynaecological cancers including cervical, endometrial and ovarian cancers.

Since these two cancer antigens were recognized a number of others have been isolated, some more useful than others.

USING MONOCLONAL ANTIBODIES TO FIND CANCER CELLS

Remarkably, scientists have known about cancer antigens since the turn of the century. But it has been only in the last twenty to thirty years that they have had the technology to put them to good use. In the last decade, the discovery of monoclonal antibodies has made the task of identifying antigens in people with cancer a great deal easier.

Monoclonal antibodies are designed to latch onto their 'mirror-image' protein antigens on the surface of the tumour cells. In theory, the technique of 'cloning' the antibodies should make available unlimited quantities of identical, highly specific antibodies ready to home in very precisely on the antigens on tumour cells. In practice, the scaling up of production of these monoclonal antibodies has not been easy and there are still shortages. But scientists believe that it is just a matter of time before the technology which has brought monoclonal antibodies will fulfil its early promise.

It is hoped that new monoclonal antibodies will really prove their worth in diagnosing secondary tumours. Established scanning methods are relatively good at finding primary tumours. Where they fall down is in detecting the small number of cancer cells which frequently evade primary treatment, such as surgery or radiotherapy, and require courses of chemotherapy to mop them up.

In some cancers, such as breast and ovarian cancers, courses of chemotherapy are given almost routinely following the initial surgery or radiotherapy. But the unpleasant side-effects of anti-cancer drugs make their use in all but the most necessary cases undesirable. So a technique which can show whether or not any cells really have escaped from the primary site and are setting up shop as metastases will be very valuable.

Flushed with the limited success of using monoclonal antibodies in diagnosis, scientists then asked themselves whether these antibodies could also be of use in the treatment of cancer.

WHAT NEXT IN TREATMENT?

A number of specialist cancer centres are now experimenting with monoclonal antibodies for the treatment of cancer. There are three main approaches.

The simplest method of treatment is to inject 'naked' monoclonal antibodies geared to binding with antigens on the surface of tumour cells. Bearing in mind that in the normal immune reaction it is the binding of defence antibodies to foreign-cell antigens which triggers the destruction of invading organisms, it was hoped that monoclonal antibodies binding to cancer antigens would trigger a similar reaction. A bit like the class sneak, the monoclonal antibody points the finger at the tumour and waits for the local 'heavies' to come and sort it out!

This approach has already been used to treat lymphomas, but it is really too early to say how well it works. Doctors are not overly optimistic that antibodies on their own can trigger the destruction of tumours. It just seems too much to hope for.

This is why some hospitals are attaching 'weapons' to the antibodies which are then allowed to act simply as the guidance system for the missiles. The weapons fall into two groups: radioactive isotopes and drugs.

The radioactive isotopes are similar to those used in diagnosis. For example, an isotope iodine 131 emits both beta and gamma rays. The gamma rays are used for monitoring the tumour and the beta rays for actually destroying the tumour cells. This isotope has been used to treat both bowel tumours and neuroblastoma. People have responded to the treatment, but it is far too early to say whether there are significant advantages over other forms of treatment.

The same is true for the third option. This involves tagging the monoclonal antibodies to anti-cancer drugs. A number of well-established drugs are being used and it is hoped that by enabling the drugs to be more specific in the cells which they attack there will be fewer side-effects of treatment and higher doses of the drugs will get to the target tumours. As well as standard anti-cancer drugs, doctors are also using toxins, such as ricin – the so-called 'umbrella' poison since it was used to kill a Bulgarian journalist six years ago when it was concealed in the tip of an umbrella.

All of these approaches using monoclonal antibodies to target therapy will remain experimental for some years and only small numbers of people will be given the treatment in the course of clinical trials. There is a good deal of optimism, but cancer specialists have seen more than their fair share of wonder drugs sink without trace. And for the foreseeable future the vast majority of people with cancer will have to rely on step-by-step improvements of tried and tested methods of treatment.

At a recent meeting of one of the research organizations looking for new anti-cancer drugs, delegates heard how only a handful of the hundreds of new drugs tested on people with cancer has shown any benefits. Many of these products would have seemed highly promising during animal studies but have failed to live up to expectations once they were given to humans. Unfortunately, animal tumours frequently bear little resemblance to human cancers in their reactions to drugs, and time and time again drug companies which are developing them are disappointed.

None of the new anti-cancer drugs likely to come onto the market within the next few years will be miracle cures. They may have fewer side-effects and they may have significant advantages for specific cancers; but they will not be blanket cures for all types of cancer.

GETTING THE IMMUNE SYSTEM TO FIGHT BACK

The idea of developing drugs which will boost the body's immune system into destroying tumours has been a goal of cancer researchers for years. It would be the ideal solution and throughout the 1970s there were lengthy sessions on 'immunotherapy' at every cancer conference. Why, researchers kept asking themselves, if the immune system can overcome numerous invading organisms does it not recognize tumours as foreign and destroy them too? There is also some indirect evidence that from time to time the body does get rid of tumours on its own. People who die in road accidents and from causes other than cancer, for example, are found to have tumours which have clearly caused no symptoms. And it is thought that some tumours mysteriously disappear without their owner ever knowing they were there. This would tie in with the fact that a small proportion of tumours do regress for no obvious reason.

For years, doctors have tried to identify and harness the 'middle men' of the immune system – the substances which stimulate immune cells into action. One well-known group of drugs which appears to have this function is the interferons. And more recently has come the discovery of another family, the interleukins.

Since the body makes its own interferons and interleukins the idea of using them in treatment is to boost the body's natural supplies to make them trigger an attack on the tumour. The problem lies in the fact that there appears to be a world of difference between the body using its own interleukins and coping with massive extra amounts from outside. In some studies people have reacted very badly to the interleukins and required days of intensive care to get back on their feet. This has been disappointing but does not mean that there is no future for interleukins and other similar substances. It simply means that it will probably take longer than expected to find the proper place in treatment for these substances.

What has helped complicate matters is the fact that many of the immune 'middle men', generally referred to collectively as lymphokines, of which the interleukins are simply one group, have been discovered separately and almost simultaneously by different groups of scientists around the world. Thus one chemical frequently has several different names so it may seem that this week there are six potential cures for cancer when in fact there is only one and even that is not quite as exciting as originally thought!

These new approaches to cancer treatment, though novel in the fact that they aim to boost the immune system into defending itself against cancer, still suffer from the basic drawback that they are trying to correct something that has already gone wrong; the tumour is already there.

The last and perhaps longest term approach to cancer therapy of the future lies with the oncogenes – those tiny pieces of DNA (deoxyribonucleic acid) which, when inappropriately switched on or off, seem able to turn a normal cell into a cancerous one. If only scientists could find out what determines the control of these genes they believe that they could interfere with those badly behaved genes which seem to trigger cancer.

In the short term the most they can hope to do is to block the products of these genes – the growth factors which seem to play a role in tumour cells dividing out of control. But this can only be an interim measure. If they are really to get to the heart of the matter they must be masters of the oncogenes.

TOWARDS GREATER AWARENESS

New, more effective ways of treating and eventually of preventing cancer will be vital to future generations. But equally important will be a more caring approach to the day-to-day problems encountered not only by people with cancer but also by their friends and relatives.

The more enlightened medical teams looking after people with cancer do realize that treatment is not just about destroying tumours; it is also about relieving emotional distress and about making life comfortable for people with cancer whether they have many years to live or just a few days.

We, the consumers, can do much to help ourselves. By making an effort to understand the options which are open to us and discussing them with those close to us we can feel less helpless and more able to cope with what is inevitably a time of great upheaval.

There is a growing network of support groups, both nationally and locally, which can provide well-informed help and advice and the opportunity to meet others in a similar situation. At last, families and friends are being included more openly in discussions and decisions which are likely to affect them almost as much as those with cancer.

There is still a long way to go. Cancer is not yet out of the closet. And people still find it hard to talk about it – as we found when we were researching this book. But progress is being made and it is to be hoped that those future generations who get cancer will at least be spared some of the fear and frustration, the lack of information and understanding frequently suffered by their parents and grandparents.

FURTHER READING

Gidske Anderson, *It Happened to Me*, Futura, 1986
Penny Brohn, *Gentle Giants*, Century, 1986
Bob Champion and Jonathan Powell, *Champion's Story*, Gollancz, 1981
Jory Graham, *In the Company of Others*, Gollancz, 1983
Wendy Green, *The Long Road Home*, Lion, 1985
Ethel Helman, *An Autumn Life*, Faber & Faber, 1986
Richard Lamerton, *Care of the Dying*, Penguin, 1980
Richard Lamerton, *East End Doc*, Lutterworth, 1986
Christine Piff, *Let's Face It*, Gollancz, 1985

INDEX